Change It!

8 Steps to Create Positive
TRANSFORMATION
in Your
Health,
Relationships
& Income

C.J. ALEXANDER

WOW Book Publishing™

First Edition Published by C.J. Alexander

Copyright ©2018 C.J. Alexander

WOW Book Publishing™

Editor: Gill Prior
www.prioredting.co.uk
info@prioredting.co.uk
Editor & Formatter:
fiverr.com/amazing_writing

Paperback ISBN: 978-1-7311-9986-7

First Edition, December 2018

Dedication

This book is dedicated to you, the reader. I would like to thank you personally for taking the time to invest in yourself. Hopefully, reading this will allow you to make positive changes in your life.

The content in this special book has been taken from the very best concepts and strategies that I have discovered and learned over the last few years, taken from some of the world's experts in the field of self-transformation. This sought-out knowledge has been transformed into this book, along with the guidance of the award-winning author, Vishal Morjaria. I would like to share this knowledge with you, so that you can begin an incredible journey of positive transformation through any of the major challenges in your life.

Regards

C.J. Alexander
(Chris James Alexander)

Contents

About the Author

C.J. Alexander wrote this book for you to make some necessary decisions that will enable positive change in your life.

C.J. changed his life in his late twenties, by turning a discouraging and devastating period into a learning experience at the age of thirty-three. The loss of his best friend, followed by a chain of downward spiralling events, led to a saga of ongoing depression and severe stress heading towards suicide. This experience left a detrimental but significant impact on his life. It brought a tremendous amount of pain, pressure and devastation. However, the support of professional help and self-development enabled his transformation for a new life, including better health, positive relationships, new career and diverse opportunities for income, all within three years! This then became a large involvement for astonishing knowledge and wisdom, to empower others who have been through similar experiences.

The author currently lives in the UK, and enjoys travelling, learning and experiencing the best concepts and philosophies of personal development. The information in this book has been influenced by some of the best sources in the world, with secrets to success in life. The aim of this book is to help you make positive transformations in your life, by allowing you to shift your mindset into a new self-belief system, to achieve things that could allow a more prosperous way of living.

C.J. has developed an extraordinary philosophy of life that is oblivious to most of us. Many times, he has been challenged but rather than being swallowed up by those challenges, he has taken the learnings and implemented them to create a better future. These findings have been inspired by some of the world's most influential experts, such as the late Jim Rohn, John Asaraf, Tony Robbins, Bob Proctor, Les Brown, Tai Lopez and mentor Vishal Morjaria.

By sharing these simple yet effective thought processes with others in need for change, C.J. has helped many people to kick start their thinking and action process to succeed positively in life. The process of creating positive change isn't really all that complicated. All you have to do is sit back, read and absorb some of the profound knowledge.

Then, begin to apply it to your own life. Taking action is the key if you wish to reap the rewards and useful results that will positively change your life forever.

Acknowledgements

I would like to express a special thanks to my beautiful daughter, who has been a huge inspiration for me to make changes in my health, relationships and income, which also enabled me to apply those experiences and knowledge to write this book. She has been my source of inspiration and motivation since the day she was born to always strive for excellence and become the best person I could be, not only to provide for her, but to also instil in her the great philosophies of life, and hope that someday, she will create her own legacy.

Thanks to my very good friend J. Chambers for his wisdom on the power of Goal Setting and Law of Attraction. These concepts were shared with me to start a revolutionary journey to implement positive change in my life and the lives of others. I thank you J, for your wisdom, beliefs and faith in me. A special thank you to my late best friend D.P Auluck, who guided me through various turning points in my adult life. RIP and God bless your soul.

A special thanks to my close family and friends, for being there and supporting me throughout my journey so far. A special thanks to my mother who has raised me to always support and help others. Also, my Dad for the financial support and teachings on the value of money and investment, during recent years.

Some of the greatest discoveries along this journey were the great philosophies by one of the world's most influential thought leaders of our time, Mr. Jim Rohn whom I rated as the ultimate master teacher and mentor of personal development. Those who want to continue to develop their skills and philosophies should hear and absorb his astonishing words of wisdom to become successful. I also want to acknowledge the influences of John Asaraf, the founder of Neurogym and Les Brown, a profound motivational speaker.

The above experts have dedicated their lives towards helping people achieve a better belief system, so it is possible to become the person you truly desire to be. If you learn, study and apply these new-found strategies, you could well be on your way to achieve your goals and fulfil your dreams.

"If you want to have more, you must first become more. Success is not a doing process, it's a becoming process. Therefore, we must work harder on ourselves more than anything else."

—Jim Rohn

Testimonials

"If you are seeking positive transformation, then it is imperative that you read this book. Chris is a real pro at encouraging and supporting others to bring the best out of them. His new-found philosophies are out of this world."

—Vishal Morjaria,
Award Winning Author and International Speaker

"Some speak a lot whilst others speak very little, and then there's Chris who speaks absolute sense, genius! His insights, along with professional expertise and passion touch the minds of those that wish to grow and flourish. This book is a must read!"

—Eileen Davies-McCotter,
Transformational Life Coach

"Chris has guided me along my journey, revealing an unrestricted belief in myself. He has helped me to identify and develop areas of my life, where opportunities now feel limitless. Thank you."

—Jory Chambers,
Personal Trainer & Healthy Foods Expert

"Chris has literally changed my life! His teachings and coaching have allowed me to discover my true potential in my personal life and in business. An inspiration to us all."

—Lynsey Byers,
Events & Hospitality Manager and Mum of Two

"Chris has inspired me to be the best version of myself. His wealth of knowledge and understanding of self-development is elevating. By sharing his own life experiences, I was able to implement the foundations to transform my life."

—Lucy Curtis,
Internal Account Manager and Mum of Four

"After an accident at work, which brought devastation and trauma to my life, I turned to Chris for guidance and support. He helped me to clarify the core issues to make positive change. His philosophy is amazing!"

—Leon Dahouchi,
Construction Worker and Father of One

INTRODUCTION

Breaking Point at 80 Miles Per Hour!

Why can't I focus on this road? There are multiple flash visions in front of my eyes. Nothing but negative thoughts are going through my mind. I can't control them. I feel like I'm being dragged through a black hole. "I am losing my mind!"

While facing this battle of my sanity, I was trying to keep in the centre lane on the motorway while driving at 80mph, in my blue Volkswagen saloon at 7.45am. As I drove to work, I saw a BMW 3 series flew past in the fast lane, then I saw another silver Peugeot 307 starting to overtake me. My mind was out of control. I began to lose awareness of external noises; I just can't focus because my negative thoughts had taken over. Finally, I reached my work place at about 8:12am, and I heard the school bell ring. I saw students running into their classrooms as I walked towards my form room. I looked at the floor as I dragged my feet. My palms began to sweat, my heart beats slightly faster and my chest started to wheeze. It felt like the earth was collapsing at my feet, pulling me towards the ground.

My heart was racing more, and I could control the thoughts. I heard a voice say "Good Morning!" I put on a brave face, crack a weak smile and I just carry on walking to my room. I began to feel my hands shake and my whole body started to judder every few seconds at this point. I struggled to focus, but managed to enter the room where my student form group was waiting for me.

Fast forward, I looked up at the clock and it was now 10:13am. Two hours have passed, almost two classes have been taught. I still can't shake off these dark thoughts and feelings of fear, anxiety, worry, stress, confusion and panic. I felt like I was going insane. I began to feel dazed; there was no focus or complete self-control, nothing but a sheer darkness of confusion, fear and anxiety.

I began to struggle for breath, taking fast breaths every second. It became very hot. Sweat started to pour. I started to lose balance and my students were looking at me strangely. I tried my best to gain self-control, but it becomes almost impossible . . . Then suddenly, I heard a knock at the door, it was the Assistant Head, "Excuse me sir, can I have a word please, in private." I was wanted by the Head teacher. A complaint had been made against me.

And that was it . . . the 'final blow' to the gut and to my head. I knew there and then, that was it for me. I had come to a breaking point! I felt like someone had just thrown a rock at my body and it shattered into a thousand pieces. I couldn't breathe. I felt like my life force was slowly drifting away. I tried to gather that last inner strength to stand, but I could not anymore. My vision blurred, then I saw nothing but darkness; I had blacked out.

Around 1pm, I was lying in a hospital bed, staring at the

ceiling with blurred vision. Confused, dazed and wondering how my life had reached a point of pure destruction. I didn't know who I was anymore. **But there was one thing I did know. I had to break out of this condition of imprisonment and get my life back on track.** My health, if not my life depended on it.

From the chain of bad events that had occurred over the past 20 months including, the loss of my best friend, open surgery on my baby girl, increasing financial burdens and the intense pressures of the job, had led to my first panic attack. Due to all the compounding events that had happened including the stresses, work overload and inner fears that were taking place in my mind, I had finally hit the breaking point. I was completely burned out.

I knew at that point, I had ENOUGH! With my career, personal relationships and unstable well-being. I said, "NO MORE!" I'm in need of a change in my life, no matter what it takes!

A 'Quantum Leap' defined:
'The explosive jump that was made,
moving from one place to another.'

STEP 1

Chance: Understanding YOU

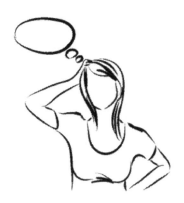

YOU at This Precise Moment

At this precise moment in time, what are you experiencing? Are you in a happy place? Or are you feeling discouraged? Do you feel that you require more in life? Do you feel content, but you know there is more out there for you? Or you just don't know what you want in life but understand there is a chance that you want to do something better? What is holding you back from becoming truly happy?

Well, if you feel that you can relate to any of the above, then I have a good news for you. If you wish to create a positive change, you must first find out what it is that you want. I mean, what you REALLY want in life, and find a way of making it happen. We all go through difficult times, through the struggles and the complexities of life. But you've got to be a good planner and a good dreamer to achieve more. Most of all, you must take a chance. If you don't take a chance, how will you ever know what's possible for you? You will stay stuck in the same place, repeating life patterns over and over again. The definition of insanity is to continue to do the same thing, but expect a different result. In all honesty, you must take a chance, and you have to make some changes in order to make things work for you. There's a whole wide world out there with amazing opportunities. Wherever you are in life, there is always a chance that you can make things work for you to create a better lifestyle. In this world, we only get one life; you have to make the most of it.

If this is somewhat difficult to acknowledge and digest, then I highly recommend that you consider a new philosophy on what you make of life. To assist in this new concept of thought processing, the *Challenge to Succeed* audio programme by Jim Rohn will reveal secrets and interesting truths; an invaluable source of new information.

What Do YOU Want?

What is it that you really want? Decide today (not tomorrow) on what you really want, because the universe will only give you what you ask for. If you ask for vague things, you will end up with vague results. The key is to decide on exactly what you really want. Be crystal clear, take action towards the goal, and you will begin to see this start to manifest.

I will give you an example. Have you ever thought about that particular car that you perhaps wanted or the expensive fashion designer piece you desired? Or a phone, laptop, or watch? These materialistic things you desired and subconsciously ask for, (before you even know it) are already in your possession. Now, I'm not saying that you would say "Oh, I want that," and then walk into a store and buy it, regarless of the cost, but with subconscious thinking and manifestation of obsession, you will find a way. That is the power of deciding on what you want, and then attracting it to yourself.

Some may call this the 'The Law of Attraction'; however, I often refer to it as 'being obsessed with your goals and dreams, and working your butt off to achieve them.' I will cover this area in detail later in this book. My philosophy on achieving what you want is to write down at least five things that you really want and then turn them into five goals. These goals will help you move towards where you want to be. I'm not talking about things that you could easily do in a year, I'm talking about things that will move you forward in your life that are going to create transformation. They can be as crazy as you like or as big as you like, but it has to be something that's going to make a positive change in your life. You must focus on these goals consistently (not constantly) and work hard to reach them.

Prosperity Pyramid

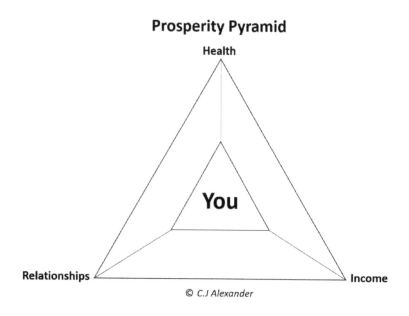

Health

You

Relationships

Income

© C.J Alexander

The Prosperity Pyramid

In life, there are three elements that we focus on as human beings. The first element (and utmost important) is our *health and survival.* We must take good care of our health. If we don't have good health, then what do we have? The second element is our *relationships,* who we associate ourselves with and our loved ones. The third element is our *income.* How do we generate income? How are we able to pay our bills? How do we support our families? How do we pay for luxuries? This all boils down to income.

The three elements aligned together make up what I like to call the '*Prosperity Pyramid.*' In fact, there is actually one more element, and that element is *YOU.* Now that you are aware of the elements of the Prosperity Pyramid, I would like you to think about how you want your health to be? How you want your relationships to be? And what type of income you want?

Identify where you are right now in each of the three elements, then think about what you can do to move forward. YOUR life is the most significant, which you might mistake for your family, your friends or your children, but in reality, it is YOU. If you don't take care of you, then who is going to? If you aim to get those three elements right in your life, I guarantee you will transform your life and become a truly prosperous person, in your health, relationships and income.

Choice

The majority of a person's lifetime boils down to choice. Yes, that's right, you are where you are today due to the choices you have made in the past. Every single decision you make in your life has been down to pure choice. From the job you decided to take, to that business deal, and the relationships that you were in, to the health choices that you have made or the intake of food and drink that you consume. It is all down to choice. If you break it down and work out how many choices you've actually made in your life, you would be astonished to discover all the decisions you've made that have brought you to this point in life.

Now we all have to make decisions (period!) some are good, while some turn out to be bad. The point is, whether they turn out to be good or bad, you learn from them. You must take whatever choices you have made in the past as experiences, because you can only learn from them, NOT dwell on them.

My point is, now you have a choice; you have choices of what directions you want your life to go. Irrespective of what others have told you otherwise, or those who always assume they know what's best for you, IT IS NOT their life. This is your life! You always have the choice, and you deserve a great life. So, why not make it a great one. Why not make those choices for yourself? Why not stand up and say "You know what... I'm going to do this for ME and no one else."

Some people may think you are being selfish. Well, you know what . . . whatever opinion someone has of you, that is their business, not yours. Remember, the choice is yours. You can either decide to do what you want and leap into fear, or you can just continue to make repetitive choices, based on someone else's assumptions, which lead you to become paralysed by fear and inability to move out of your comfort zone.

How Did You Get to This Point?

If you think about it, from the day you were born, you were brought into this world being completely dependent on your parents or guardians to raise you. When you got to about the age of three, you probably started to make your own choices about what you did want and didn't want.

When you reached your school years, you were instructed by teachers and educators, and also often given strict instructions by your parents or guardians. Discipline was enforced a lot more at this point. This is when your programming of the world started and your personality began to develop. From when you were first born, you had what's called an inner child persona, where you were carefree. No great fears in the world. Just exploring things because you wanted to do them.

But as you got older and you grew into society, those around told you what's good and not good for you. What you should do, what you can't do and what journeys you should take in life; from there, it just spirals out of control, with the influences that are around you.

After high school, you perhaps went on to college or a work-based internship. If you did continue with further education, you would have gone on to university, and then after that ultimately got a job. My point is, where did it all come from? Who told you to take that route? Is it because everybody around you was doing that and you just followed the crowd? Or have you had that inner instinct to do something greater? Let's face it, why try to fit in, when you were born to stand out?

So, let's just take a minute. Look back and think about how you've got to this point, because the reality is (without being too blunt) that you have got to this point in life because of the choices that you've made. Almost everything that's happening in your life today is down to the choices made.

I'm sorry to say it so bluntly, but unfortunately that is the case. This is not entirely your fault, there are various combinations of factors that are down to the influences of society. Lucky for you, you can take a chance TODAY and change things. Move on to the things that YOU want to do. Change can be very scary (I know) but I guarantee somewhere along the line that things will work out for you, which will lead onto a better area of life.

Faith

Faith has got to be one of the most powerful spiritual energies that you can have on this earth. If you truly believe and have faith in something, eventually it will manifest into your desires.

Now, I'm not saying you should just rely on hope; as hope is like a weak prayer. You've got to have true faith in yourself and what it is you're looking for. I've had many times where I've had faith in myself, when I knew I could do something great, but it was difficult to act upon due to the circumstances. However, there is always a way of getting to where you need to be.

My point is that 'inner strong faith' can draw you towards what you want, and it can completely change your perception of how you feel about yourself or any other beliefs that you have. You've got to have faith, especially in yourself, to move forward and become that person you wish to be. It is a powerful spiritual tool to use which will get you through life, especially when you think all hope is lost.

The chances are, if you lose faith, you will lose the will to continue. But if you truly know deep down that there's a way to move forward, you are more likely to achieve it. Just keep strong in faith. Keep working towards what you want, whether it is, a new job or a new career, a business idea that you want to get off the ground, a fitness or weight goal, or perhaps a new start with a relationship. Along with faith, you've got to work hard towards whatever it is you desire. Continue to get up every day, have faith and work towards your goals of where you want to be.

There Is Always a Better Way

No matter what circumstances you are in now, on the other side there is triumph. It doesn't matter how deep down in the dumps you are or how long your problems have been going on, there is always a better way. The key is to never give up; just keep trying. There are many people throughout history who have considered giving up. If you look at some of the biggest successes in the world today, they were not an overnight success. They had to work towards it, to make sure it's going to work. Sooner or later with persistence, consistency, faith, they managed to pull it off and now they have changed the world.

Entrepreneurs such as Steve Jobs of Apple Inc., Thomas Edison who invented the light bulb, Bill Gates with Microsoft computer software, along with many other successful people in the world have gone through many trials on their journeys, but have worked through it and managed to pull through. On August 28th 1963, Martin Luther King Jr. delivered one of the most inspirational speeches of all time, in which he had a dream that black and white people could co-exist together in society; the rest is history. Just take a look at the world now. If one person can have a vision to change the world, I think that you can make a better way for yourself. It is possible!

The Fear and the Leap

In life, deep down, we want to do more. We want to try but we just fear doing anything about it. More so, it is the fear of the challenge, the fear of rejection, the fear of failure, the fear that you're just going to end up back at square one. For most, they fear the change itself. If you don't try, then there will be no different outcome. There is no change. There is no new result. So, you have to take a leap of faith and jump right into the fear - just do it, because I promise there is always a better way.

Fear is often referred to as 'False Experiences Appearing Real.' About 90 percent of the things that we worry about never happen. It might feel rocky, it might feel tough at first, but taking action will work out for you in the long run. You must be able to take that fear and leap right into it. You will learn so much more by taking that initial leap of faith. It is like the sayings, "sink or swim" or "fight or flight." One of the ways to start the process of overcoming fear is to read books. There is a great book called *Feel the Fear and Do It Anyway,* by Susan Jeffers, which will give you a new outlook on what is possible, explaining how fear is all in the mind.

We all have fears. Fear is just a fragment of what's going on in our minds. Danger is very real, so in order to survive, we have to protect ourselves, but if you can conquer that fear, you can achieve anything. Entrepreneur and star of the movie *The Secret*, T. Harv Eker, stated that "Nothing has meaning other than the meaning you give it." Basically, that means whatever you are giving attention to in your mind will multiply your thoughts. Therefore, if you can conquer that in your mind, you can focus more on what you want, rather than what you don't want.

Thoughts DO become things. The more you try to focus and block out all the junks that you don't really need to think about, the more you can grow further and faster. You need to do what's right for you, and take a leap of faith. Take something useful from this chapter, and perhaps implement it in an area that is required. My message to you is to just do what is right in your heart.

The biggest breakthroughs typically come when you're feeling the most frustrated and stuck, that's often when people make the decision to change and move forward. Most people who don't fail in life are those that never try. When you fail, don't automatically assume that you're a failure. Instead, embrace each failure as a small set back, and an opportunity to learn something new. When you move forward, you will see that it was all worth it. Take a chance. Often failures can actually be leading you further towards your goal, which is apparent only an hindsight when you get there.

Learn some simple steps on how you can make
breakthrough by taking a chance,
visit www.changeitbook.com

STEP 2

Health:
Your Health Is
Number One

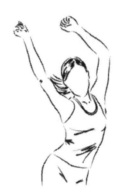

Rule Number One:

Take vital care of your health; physically, emotionally and most of all mentally. The Prosperity Pyramid that I talked about in the previous chapter includes the most valuable element - health.

If you don't have good health in life; then, what do you have? We must take care of our health. We now live in a world where technology is forever growing and society is becoming more fast paced. The stress and intensity of living are becoming a real burden for some, and as a result, we take less care of our bodies and minds.

This accounts for what we're feeding into our minds and bodies, and how our spiritual faith is developing or decreasing.

I know that there are many people in this world who are suffering through health, whether it is mental, physical, or emotional which needs healing. To avoid this suffering, we must take absolute care of ourselves. To prevent more suffering, the key is to acknowledge it, being more proactive as opposed to reactive when the suffering occurs. This can be helped by learning and training your mind to cope with stress and anxiety, focussing on body nutrition, and growing stronger in your faith and self-belief. All the above will contribute to moving you forward, but if you neglect to take care of yourself, then guess what's going to happen, you are just going to end up feeling low and discouraged, perhaps even depressed. Our health is number one. Fact!

Throughout this chapter, there will be some tips and strategies on how to work on your health. My overall number one rule is 'look after yourself.' Do what is right for you, don't take on too much or you will burn out. On the flipside of this, it is important not to neglect what you should be doing for the better. There must be a balance in your lifestyle, that will allow you to grow positively.

What Are You Consuming?

There are many things in the society that we feel can make us feel good, but what impact are they actually having in the long term? For some, this might be watching several hours of TV a day, including the news and listening to the radio. There is nothing wrong with consuming some media; however, if too much is consumed, it could be having a detrimental effect on your way of life.

We also take in what our family and friends are discussing, including the latest social topic or gossip. Even in the workplace, "Did you know?", "So and so said this." "So and so did that."

What are you reading? What type of newspaper headlines do you pay attention to? Are they positive and beneficial to you? The chances are that most are unlikely to be. So, the question is, "What are you feeding your minds?" because that will determine the outcome of what's going on in your life right now. Whatever you pour in, you are more likely to pour out.

Ask yourself, "Is this something that I want to continue to be exposed to?" "Is this good for me?" If the answer is no, then you need to change it. Set some new habits that you want to build into your lifestyle and be committed to them. Identify the junks that you are consuming and change them.

If you don't like what's in the news or on the TV, then perhaps find a good book to read or find a new hobby. Go for a walk. Get some exercises. Start writing down some notes or things that you want to do. Block out time to spend with your kids. Do some research on the internet and search for things that you are interested in. Be creative to find a way of moving forward from the old you. Yes, we do get stuck for time, but if you plan and structure your week and eliminate the unnecessary things, I'm sure you can make some time.

There is always a way to a better lifestyle. You've just got to figure out what path you want to take.

Once you have decided to create a change, be very wary of who you are around in the process. Are there people in your life holding you back? Are there certain voices that you're just sick and tired of listening to? Do you want to change your social environment? Maybe it is time to take a look into this area.

Firstly, investigate and identify what you are consuming on a daily basis, because a year, two years, five years or ten years down the line, your future could be the same as it is now, if there are no changes. Think about it. Ask yourself. "If I continue this journey, where will I be in the next five to ten years? In the blink of an eye, time will pass. The question is will you be faced with prosperity or faced with devastation and regret?

How Do You Want Your Health to Be?

What do you want your health to look like? How do you want to feel? How do you want to look? It is very important to identify this and write it down. Make a list of the top areas you would like to develop. Possibly create a vision board to view this on a daily basis to support your subconscious through visualisation.

Write down two points, (Point A) 'where you are now,' and (Point B) 'where you want to be.' Along with this, add an action plan, timescale and deadlines to help you measure the progress of your journey. There's a great book by Jack Canfield called *The Success Principles: How to Get from Where You Are to Where You Want to Be.* It is a fantastic book (which is also available on audio) that has tips on goal setting and action plans.

Where do you want to see yourself in the next six months or a year? For example, do you want to start to train and work out at the beginning of the year, ready for the summer? Everybody wants to get in shape for that beach body, to look great and feel great. This demonstrates visualisation, determination, commitment and discipline to work on your health and well-being. So, why not apply the same principles in an area of your life. In your social life, emotional well-being, physical well-being, or spiritual well-being, a goal is crucial to work towards. The quicker you work towards the goal, the sooner or later (if consistent) the transformation process will happen.

Imagine what it is going to feel like, mind, body and soul, once you start to take action. There's no point moaning about it, that will do NOTHING to move you forward. Just take some action, seek advice, research online, talk to a doctor if necessary. Maybe take some time out from work to reflect on things and start creating a healthy plan.

What Impact Is Your Life Having Right Now?

Take a look at everything that's going on around you right now, with your career, family, friends or maybe financial situations; what impact is it having on you? How do you feel? Do you feel great? So-so? or discouraged? Do you want to do something about it but feel helpless? Many of you will be experiencing similar feelings, so try to understand your pain right now, whatever the situation.

Know that there is a way to change it, just keep moving

forward, and know that by relying on faith you can move into a better position in your life. What is surrounding you that is making you unhappy? What is perhaps making you feel the way you do? What is it that you need to improve, that will have a positive impact in every area of your life? There's no better feeling in the world than the feeling of excitement, happiness, joyfulness, peace, and gratitude. Just be honest, think about what impacts your life negatively; dig deep and identify the cause.

Perhaps, you may need to talk to someone trustworthy or a trained specialist about this. There are so many therapists and counsellors out there, who can help you. You can even find support in one of the many social media community groups. Talking to someone, especially somebody you don't really know, can make such a difference. It can reveal the truth patterns on your life, which could allow some changes for the better.

Are You Living in the Moment?

There are a lot of people out there who say, "Once I do this, then I will be happy," "If I earn more money, then I will be happy," "When I get to that point, I know I will be happy." But what is stopping you from being happy right now??? There may be things that are pulling you down because of major concerns, they may be financial burdens that you are carrying, perhaps some debts that are always behind your mind. Perhaps somebody is unhappy with you or you're unhappy with them; or a relationship that's holding you back, rather than moving you forward. Anyone of these can be a strenuous burden to you. Even with these burdens in life, you can try to be in the moment, and think of the things that make you the happiest person, just for that split second. Find the happiness in what you have, and try not to compare yourself to the other person. Just for a split second, think of what life would be like if these burdens were to disappear and things fell into place the way you wanted them to.

If you can do this, maybe you are able to increase the moments to a few more seconds, then scale it up to a minute, five minutes, ten minutes and more. By applying this into a daily routine while focusing on what you really want, you can find a sense of happiness each time. Just by achieving this slight shift in your thought patterns, you will be able to focus more on optimism. As this develops over time, and the areas in your life start to improve (health, relationships and income) you would have expanded that tiny feeling of 'being in the moment' and transformed it into a new more permanent reality. Imagine, waking up every day and dancing out of bed because you love what you do, and your life is how it should be. Imagine that! Well here's the thing, there are many people out there who are already applying this technique and seeing such results. Whether they are successful, wealthy or non-wealthy, being content and happy is what really counts.

Try and live in the moment, even if it is only for a few seconds. The positive feeling may grow into a minute, then possibly into a new reality. If you decide to try this, find something that makes you really happy from the heart. It might be spending time with your loved ones, socialising with friends, travelling, a trip to the beach, being creative or a sense of achievement. Seek to find what makes you truly happy, and live it in the moment.

What Emotions Are You Feeling?

Emotions can determine a lot of our decisions, based on how we feel. If we feel really happy, we can make one type of decision, but if we feel unhappy with low moods, then we often tend to make different decisions. Emotions can ultimately have consequences, based on the decisions we make. So, we must be in tune with our emotions and master them to avoid the chances of a negative impact on our lives. On the other hand, there may be opportunities where you need to act fast. If you decide to take immediate action, you can only learn from it, whether it turns out to be a good or bad decision.

Emotions can either move us forward or can hold us back, becoming a prisoner in the mind, but if you continue to work on them to move forward, and learn how to tackle them when you feel challenged, you will find a way of managing your emotions. If you achieve this, you could be happier in your relationships, financial situations and health.

From having experienced difficulties with my own state of mind, this had a massive impact on my emotions, which then impacted my body and other areas of my life at the time. Emotions can really dictate some of our actions, as a result, if you can control them and not rise to the negative aspects, they can be replaced with more positive emotions. For example, if someone says something to you that you find offensive and you react to it in a negative way (based on your emotions) it could have an adverse impact. However, if you know how to control your emotions and maybe let things go quicker, the result from your reaction to the same situation could be much more beneficial to you, or at least not have the same negative connotations.

Here's a quick exercise that you could do to help you. If you're struggling with your emotions, just take a minute in a quiet spot to try and let go of EVERYTHING. Be in the moment and truly believe that things will work out for you. Be at peace, control your emotions, take one DEEP breath and exhale. Try this technique and see if it works for you.

Health versus Wealth

Most people in the world believe that in order to have a good health, you need to be wealthy. This can be true in some cases; however, this is not a concrete fact. As I have said in this chapter, you can be in the moment to produce a good state of mind. You have the options to take care of your body, mind and spirit. So, you don't necessarily have to retain a lot of money to have good health.

You can be in a place of prosperity right now, where your mind and your body are working together in a healthy state. It is all down to the conditions of your situation and how you feel. If you eat right, exercise and feed your mind with information that you find positive, this can allow you to tune in to your spirit. Mediation, yoga, spiritual practices or talking to a friend who won't judge you, are great ways to lift your mental state without investing a huge amount of money. The contributing factors of a positive shift in the mind tend to come from talking to people within an encouraging community group.

You may also want to seek guidance on how you can work on your income, which could well be the cause of your health problems; however, you don't always have to confuse money with health solution because it is not always the case.

I believe if you really want to be healthy, you can be healthy, but it starts from the mind. Act upon it and have unlimited faith that you can turn things around along with the right support. Give it time and seek advice if necessary, to help you improve your health.

Decide on Your Well-Being Today

You have the opportunity to do amazing things in this world. You have a world of resources out there, especially with advancements of the internet and the number of books available. Today, we live in an information age, and with the invaluable knowledge that is out there, you can transform your well-being for the better. There are so many books out there that are highly resourceful, along with thousands of audio books to choose from. The world is full of useful information that can help you, you've just got to seek it.

However, it can be difficult in some situations, going through the tough times. Especially when you're feeling low and struggle to improve your situation. You've just got to say to yourself (with unstoppable belief) that things WILL change for the better, and everything is working out for you, along with the subconscious thoughts of self-determined action. Once you achieve a slight shift in mindset, you will begin to see the world from a place where things can get better. There is a great possibility you will even move towards feeling prosperous, but you've got to tell yourself that, and have unlimited faith in yourself to be able to do that.

One of the things I would suggest to reduce daily stress and anxiety, and even depression, is to meditate every day to support your well-being. There is a vast array of proof on the beneficial effects of meditation for the mind and ultimately the body, should you chose to further research the topic. Also, seek the right vitamins, the right foods and nutrients to aid your progress. Exercise is also very important on a daily or weekly basis, even short walks can have a huge impact. By taking a deep breath every now and then, and visualizing how your well-being should be, this can be a supplier to increase serotonin levels over time. *(Serotonin is a neurotransmitter of the brain, popularly thought to be a high contributor to feelings of well-being and happiness.)*

Remember, your health is number one! Once you get that right, then you will be on your way to living a more prosperous healthy life. John Asaraf, the founder of *Neurogym* has a phenomenal 'brain training' programme called 'Innercise,' which provides ground-breaking strategies and coping mechanisms, which can help empower the mind to transform your well-being. I would recommend trying 'Innercising' to start the development process. These videos can be found on YouTube.

To learn how you can develop a healthy mind with
a simple guide, visit www.changeitbook.com

STEP 3

Aspire:
You Deserve More

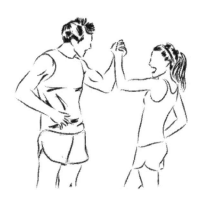

Want More? Just Ask

Have you heard of the 'Law of Attraction?' If you have, great! If you haven't, I will cover this later on in this book. The Law of Attraction in its simple form, is asking for what you truly want and believing that you will receive it to bring about the physical change in your life through manifestation. However, you can't just kick back and say "I want..," and then expect it to turn up the next day. I mean, really ask for what's in your heart and be in tune in with your spirit. If this is done with true belief and faith, things will turn around in no time. This is a tough theory to grasp, but that is just the way the world is.

Those who are spiritually in tune with their mind, body and spirit can ask for things that they want, focus on it, work towards it and eventually it will show up. Now, I am not a master at this, but I do know people who have done this and have become happy and successful in what they do. The most common reasons some people struggle to manifest what they want are; they haven't given it enough thought or focus or they don't know what they truly want. Throughout this book, I will cover the methods on this retained by mentors who are experts in this field.

For anything to work, you must be consistent. Bruce Lee once said, "I don't fear the man that can do a thousand kicks. I fear the man that can do one kick for a thousand days." Wow! To echo this incredible quote, consistency is the key long term rather than expecting immediate results. By asking and believing in the possibility for change, you are allowing your faith to grow. Just Ask! To start, just look to the sky and ask for what it is that you want. That's it! Find a way of working towards your desire and eventually you will start to see the results before you know it.

Life Balance Circle: Time for Change

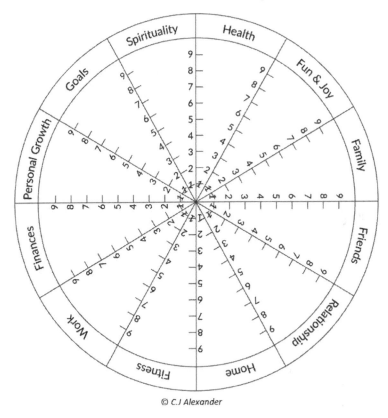

© C.J Alexander

Challenge:

Step 1

1. Use the life balance circle to evaluate the different aspects of your life.

2. On a scale of 1-10 (1 being the lowest and 10 being the highest), circle how satisfied you are with each

area of your life . . . Be <u>honest</u> *and go with your gut feeling.*

3. *Once completed, go around the circle and join up the numbers chosen for each life area.*

   (This will give you clarity on the areas that are going well, and the areas that need improvement)

Step 2

1. *Pick TWO areas that you really want to improve on.*

2. *Write down THREE action steps for each of the chosen areas picked.*

3. *Set some goals and actions to be taken, to work on them.*

What Are Your Goals?

Goals are the GPS to the success and outcome in your life. If you don't have goals, then there is no destination to arrive at. We all strive towards different things in our lives but, it is imperative to set goals, otherwise, there is a good chance that you will wake up one day and say "How did I get to this point?" If this is a new concept to you, then perhaps take a short break from this chapter, decide and write down the goals that could change your life for the better. If you wish to, do it today!

Here are 3 questions to ask yourself . . .

- What do I WANT?
- What do I want to CHANGE?
- WHEN do I want it to HAPPEN?

Goal setting is fundamentally the pinnacle starting point in making changes in your life. For the last few years, I have set five goals each year that I knew could make some dramatic changes in my life. From the day I decided to do it has not only changed my life but also continued to develop the person I am today.

"The greatest asset is not what you possess. The greatest asset is the person you have become."- Jim Rohn

Many successful people in the world including entrepreneurs, philanthropists and top professionals tend to use goals to progress. Nowadays, it is becoming more apparent to use goals in your daily life, which is why I want to stress the importance of goal setting. Goals can be used in many areas of your life, including losing weight, earn more money or seeking the right person that you want in your life.

New Year's resolutions and wishful thinking do not work to make significant changes in your life. As soon as January 1st comes around, you're fired up to stick to the resolutions. Research shows that around 12 days later, many people tend to give up. Here's a tip . . . Take all your New Years' resolutions and wishful thinking, screw them up and toss them in the trash! Only by setting goals will you make a difference. These are actual goals that you need to set yourself. One of the best ways to do that is to decide what you want, and what you want to change with a year. Goals must not only be achievable, they must also be realistic within a time frame. Find a way of creating these goals through written text or visuals, and really think . . . "Are they achievable? Are they realistic? Are they manageable with the time allocated?"

Another good way of looking at your goals is by visualising the 'bigger picture,' and having the end results in mind. What is it going to look like? What is it going to feel like? What will you have? By answering these questions, you will begin to build a 'visual subconsciousness' in your mind, so that you can work towards the goal. I can tell you now, this method, alongside goal setting, has been one of the best things I've done to keep me focused along the journey, to make positive transformations in my life, and to help others do the same. The magnificence of this strategy is that when you experience it and it works for you, then you can share the experience with others to help them achieve their own goals, allowing more happiness and success to spread by creating a ripple effect.

Dream Big

When you daydream and visualise your ultimate fantasy of pure abundance, it can make you feel good inside. No matter how big the dream is; anything is possible, and can be turned into your own reality. It doesn't matter how far away you think you are from the fantasy to reality, there is no limit to how big you can dream. It is your dream. There are a

lot of (so called) realists out there who will say, "What???
No, that's not achievable, you can't do that."

In this world, there are optimists and pessimists. The
definition of an optimist is, *'a person who tends to be hopeful
and confident about the future or the success of something.'*
Someone who wants to go the extra mile, break the rules of
limitations and strive for more; leading with hope and faith
for the better.

Pessimists are, *'people who tend to see the worst aspect of
things or believe that the worst will happen.'* They prefer to
keep grounded because of their belief system or their own
limitations. Notice how I said 'their own limitations.' Their
mind just can't break away from what they are too familiar
with. This is the difference between 'eye sight' and 'mind
sight.' I believe that we should be able to say to people,
"You know what? F*** It! I'm going to do this anyway. I'll do
my thing and you do yours!" Remember, the opinion from
others is their business, not yours.

If you try and it works out, brilliant. If it doesn't, just
carry on working towards achieving your goals. Don't focus
on the setback or what others will think of you. Never stop
trying until you succeed. Never give up on a dream, because
if you do, then it is over. If you continue and keep getting
back up, that's true success. Les Brown often quotes in
his motivational talks, "If you get knocked down, try to land
on your back, because if you can LOOK up, you can get UP,
you have GREATNESS in YOU."

We must dream big to aim for the lifestyle (health,
relationships and income) that we desire. I have researched
many extraordinary and successful people in this world,
who have achieved dreams they could have never imagined

were possible at first. Nevertheless, with vision (mind sight), focus and faith, you can manifest your dreams into a reality. I know people who have been absolutely 'flat broke' and today, they are living extraordinary lives, which the ordinary person with pessimism will never be able to experience. Doing extraordinary things will give you an extraordinary life; doing ordinary things will give you an ordinary life, it's as simple as that. Don't follow the crowd, create your own path! Dream big, set your goals and don't quit!

Aspire to the Vision

In our lives, we need vision to see the bigger picture. This is to build visual asset (the destination) in the back of the mind, so that we have something to aspire for and work towards (the path). It is imperative to be crystal clear on the vision, to be guided along the extraordinary journey. Vague wishes will provide you with vague results; therefore, it is better to be focused and clear or you may end up stuck on the hamster wheel. The best way I have discovered to create a vision is to meditate and visualise on it; break away from your own reality into complete dreamland. Embrace the vision by sight, hear, feel, touch and smell. Absorb as much as you can, to allow it to embed into your subconsciousness. Many like myself are visual learners, and therefore, if you are too, you will find this experience slightly easier than those that prefer to read or listen. What we see, hear and feel to build into our subconscious is extremely powerful.

To bring the vision to life, you can start by creating a vision board with images and words that can create the big picture of a positive future. A vision board can focus on a selection of key areas in your life, where you want to manifest new and exciting things. Then, you can begin to focus and work on these areas. However, that doesn't mean you have to constantly focus on the vision, as you are still required to live a daily life in the current reality that you live in.

This strategy can work for you, building upon the foundations of the vision by accomplishing each goal. If things don't work out in the way that you hoped, there could be good reason for this that will allow another door to open. Give the process time to work for you, but you must put the work in, and eventually positive things will start to show up in your life. The point I'm trying to make is that just by visualise your dream or ultimate goal, will create some positive framing for yourself, which is going to gravitate you towards better things in your life.

If you begin to feel worried that things are not heading in the right direction, which will affect the outcome, and things may not happen the way you want them to. All worrying does is make you feel anxious, steal your happiness, and take away your freedom. 95% of what we worry about never actually happens. The more positive and focused you are, with determined action on your vision and gen-uine feelings of excitement about your new future, the more likely you are going to work towards it. As I have ment- ioned in the previous chapter, you must have a sense of faith, a 'vigorous deep faith' that one day, your vision or dream will manifest into reality. Have a clear vision of what you want, and just keep working towards it, knowing that it will be worth it in the end.

Why Do You Want More?

Just think about it for a second, "why do you want more?" It is nice to know that you can have more and that you deserve more, but why do you want more? What will it bring you? Yes, more money or the most perfect partner could bring you happiness . . . but will it???

It is important to really think about this area, because this is where most people fail, assuming that their external desires will make everything glorious once achieved. By identifying the REAL reasons behind the desires, you can determine how your future is going to turn out. Everything we do is based on a reason or a motive, however, while in pursuit of the goal, vision or dream, we can become lost and sometimes forget why we set them out in the first place. When we want more, do we strive for more with good intent based on our core reasons? Or do we become disillusioned and just hope that things are just going to fall into our lap? Countless times I've heard people say, "Oh, I'm just going to wait until I win the lottery and then I'll be happy." The chances of that actually happening are very slim. In fact, its an average of 50 million to 1 of winning, so that person could be waiting a very long time to achieve happiness, that's if it ever happens. And even if they did by some extremely lucky chance, would they be truly happy in the end?

By searching deep, really deep, into why you want to create more for yourself, you can unlock your 'Why Power' – WHY do I want to achieve this? Keep digging and digging until you reach the 'emotional core' deep down, as to why want more to change your life and in some cases the ones you love most. Once you have discovered the 'inner why' to unlock your 'Why Power' you may be surprised at the direction you decide to take your life. The clearer things are, the easier it will become. The truth will set you free!

What Do You Believe You Can Achieve?

I believe that there are so many people out there who want to take a different direction in life, with hope that it can be achieved. But it is the self-belief behind it that determines whether you will achieve it or not. Many people will say, "I would like to, but I will never be able to do that," or "I would love to have that, but it is never going to happen to me."

It all starts with belief and knowing that it is going to happen at some point. If you don't believe in yourself and don't start believing in the possibilities that are out there, then it is unlikely it will happen. I was once told that our inner self belief will determine the outcome of our actions. Having inner self-belief is probably one of the most powerful assets that you can have, in terms of allowing yourself to grow and achieve what you want.

You've probably heard of the book *The Secret* by Rhonda Byrne. In the documentary movie, Dr. John Demartini stated that "whatever the mind can believe, it can achieve." The sheer source of the mind can be the driving force to manifest things into reality. Having great belief in yourself and the outcome, can be more than just rewarding, knowing that you have developed a life skill of positive transformation that most people are oblivious to. It all starts in the mind. Never let anybody tell you that you can't achieve something, because you can, with belief! If you listen to the naysayers, and dwell on their words, it will create self-doubt in your mind which will eventually lead to procrastination and then zero action, all because you've allowed the opinions of others to dictate your belief. Focus on your beliefs and BLOCK OUT the noise of others. You can achieve anything you want. I believe in you, so believe in yourself!

Aspire to Gain and to Serve

We live in a world today where we have a great desire to consume things, especially when it comes to our health, relationships and income. If we can have more, then we continue to want more. Is the gain for ourselves or do we want to gain more in order to serve and help others?

I'm a great believer in serving people because it has always been a part of my heart and soul, and at some point, the serving will be returned in your favour, "whatever you sow, you reap." The more you serve others in life with good intentions to help them achieve what they want, the more you will eventually receive what YOU want. Don't just serve and expect to receive, do it from the heart. In the Bible, *Galatians 5:14 (New International Version), states "Love your neighbour as yourself."* It is part of our natural instincts to serve and help from the heart. If you want to gain more in life that is absolutely fine, but find the balance to also serve others. The more you give, I'm sure that God and the universe at some point will eventually repay you for your good works. No Doubt!

Come on, let's face it, when you do good in this world, it feels good right? Yet still, we can become selfish and do things for our own intent (this is human behaviour). The chances are it may come around and bite you in the ass somewhere down the line (karma). By having gratitude and serving more people, I guarantee the rewards will be wonderful; you just have to recognise them. It is such a good feeling knowing that you served from the heart and were appreciated for your good works. It is so important that we try and serve as many people as we can in this world, and not for our own self-righteous gain. When you die, you can't take your assets with you, they will be left behind in this world. So, why not build the foundations of a prosperous and righteous soul that you can take onto the next life, while in pursuit of achieving what you want.

Act with Intent

When we aspire to achieve the things we want from a point of focus and clarity, we can then start to act with intent. The next questions to ask yourself are, "What is your core purpose? Who is it for? What is your intent to aspire? Why do you want to aspire for more?"

It took me a long time to figure out what it was that I really wanted, what the intent was and why I wanted to act upon it. After some deep thinking, I came to the conclusion that I had a passion and desire to really help and serve as many people as I could, to travel the world to serve and help others, and as a reward earn a very good living, so I can support my daughter and mother. That was my intent and purpose to aspire for greatness. I shall stand by this oath until the day I leave this world. Once fulfilled, it will have been the most single, powerful decision I could have ever made; to leave a legacy, and to know that

I fulfilled my purpose to help and serve people with good intent. So, ask yourself: "What is *my* intent?" "What is *my* main purpose in life?" "How can *I* utilise the experience, knowledge and skills that *I* have, to find *my* sole purpose in life?"

If you would like some help with setting goals, visit www.changeitbook.com

STEP 4

Numbers:
Know Them!

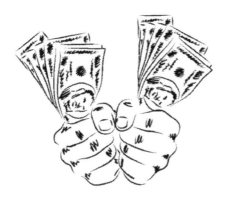

What Will It Cost You?

Before taking great action on a new journey, have a good think about the financial aspect of making a change in your life. You must consider and identify the numbers. Will this have an impact on your finances? Do you have financial backing? Will there be sacrifices that need to be made? Money is one of the biggest obstacles that we face each day. It can become an intensifying burden that produces a lot of stress for people; therefore, making changes to your circumstances can be extremely challenging. For example, if you would like to leave your job because you have just had enough, the first thing that will come to mide is "How will I survive?" or "How much can I survive on?" If you have a financial plan with some savings aside, that you can survive on, that's a good start. Nevertheless, for the majority of people this isn't an option, and so they go into panic mode, stress and severe worry states. This of course will have the opposite effect when trying to manifest your goals, only bringing about more situations which cause worry; like attracts like.

But by asking and answering a few questions on your current and future financial situation, you could be prevented from making some impulsive decisions that may have adverse consequences.

How much will this change affect my income?

How much is it going to cost me to be able to survive?

How much is it going to cost me to pursue a new journey?

What can I do to ensure the best possible result for myself?

If the answers to these questions seem daunting when you consider the life change, don't feel that this is a road block for you. There is always a possibility to make things work. If the greater part of you wants it bad enough, then you will find a way to make a breakthrough. I have made various mistakes in my time, where I have jumped into things without financially planning ahead, which caused some strain. At the end of the day, what doesn't kill us makes us stronger by learning from experiences . . . right? We do need money in order to survive; so, having a written financial plan of your income vs outgoings, is a great starting point to give you an idea for future survival.

Although, money can be a major concern when considering making changes, think of the implications in the long run, if you use money as an obstacle to prevent moving forward. Making sacrifices and changes are not the easiest of tasks but they can have a huge (positive) impact on your future. These are things to consider when weighing up the options. Don't allow the indecisive thoughts to play on your mind and cause you to procrastinate; taking action is far better than waiting too long for the right time.

Taking action towards something is far better than waiting. It has been said that taking action is worth a hundred years of thinking. With no action, there is no change. It is crucial for your own sake to think now, identify your financial position, plan ahead, take action and make steady progress.

How Much Can You Live On?

We often tend to assume that the income from a current job or business is the amount that we should live on, due to our present lifestyle. If we have high-paying jobs or business revenue, we adapted our lifestyle to suit this income. But what if you lost everything tomorrow, how much could you actually survive on?

The key is to work out what the ideal amount is that you're willing to accept to live on. Most people think they need more things to get by, including material objects and luxuries, but at the end of the day, what is more important? The materialistic things that you have now, or the sacrifices made to benefit you in the future, in terms of your well-being, your relationship and your income? Sometimes, we have to make sacrifices in order to move forward, and it can feel like you are taking a few steps back. Eventually, you will move 10 steps forward, it is just unclear to see at first. Be prepared to take that chance and have faith.

I've experienced many trials, where I have thought I had it all and everything was great, but I was never thinking about my financial position and how much I would need for a rainy day, in order to change my life. The key to a safer and less stressful future is to plan ahead and save for a rainy day, because you never know when that day might come.

Think about the essentials and how you can survive with the essentials while still being able to save for your future desired life changes. No matter how much you earn, there's always a proportion (which I will reveal later in this chapter), of how much you can put aside and how much you can actually live on. Identifying these numbers is so important. You must be able to keep track of them at all times, because 'numbers' are the name of the game in life.

What Are Your Outgoings Versus Your Income?

I know that many people work hard all month, pay their bills and then just spend, spend, and spend. As a result, they then complain halfway through the month that they've got no money left, "too much month at the end of the money." Wouldn't it be nice to have more money left than more month? It is such a nice feeling when you have money left over, but can be extremely depressing when you don't. Some people can survive on hardly anything and get through life and be happy. Some people feel that they need more; all that will do is create conflict in your mind, fabricate uncertainty, and cause worry and stress. This is just a perception of money for some; remember nothing has meaning other than the meaning you give it.

Have you ever thought about writing down all your outgoings? Just list them one by one. Write down how much is outgoing each month and at what point of the month. Therefore, you will know exactly when they are coming out of your account, how much is going out and how much is left. Then look at your income and say, "Do these outgoings match my income?" Have I got more outgoings than income?" If the answer to this is yes; then, it will be in the minus, which will lead to overdrafts, use of credit cards and loans. Whether this is a small amount or large amount, it is still a debt, 'money that you don't own' and will have to pay back. You want to be on the plus side of your account at the end of each month. See what the essential and non-essentials are. If you can do that and cut out some unnecessary things that you don't really need, those unnecessary outgoings, then could be used to build up savings or develop good investments for the long-term gain.

Maybe the reduction in outgoings could result in paying for a holiday that you want for yourself, a partner or family, perhaps a hobby that you've always wanted to try but have talked yourself out due to finances, or it could be a business venture that you have dreamed of owning.

The point is, why wait? Just get started. Don't follow the

crowd, just do something you want to do based on a solid foundation of income against the outgoings. You may hear all sorts of advice from family and friends, but it is also not always the best in terms of what you want for yourself. You have to make that choice for yourself. To reiterate, look through all your outgoings, identify the amounts and times (during the month), and cut back on the non-essentials that you don't need. Think about what you can invest in for your future.

Are You Good or Bad with Numbers?

In gambling, a lot of gamblers will keep playing because they hate to lose; unfortunately, they get hooked on the win. The adrenaline of getting that win is the drug that causes the addiction, but when they lose they feel absolutely devastated until they get their next fix with another play. Unlike gamblers, those who are successful keep track of the numbers, thus making smarter decisions when it comes to money. In casinos, they are constantly keeping track of the numbers of wins and losses several times a day to make sure that every penny is accounted for. It is imperative to use this analogy to tailor it to your own income and outgoings because if you don't, you will end up becoming oblivious to where your money has gone at the end of every month. It is not a matter of how much money you make, but how much money you keep!

Being generous with money is a good thing, but if you become an over giver without keeping track of the numbers your bank account will feel it. Discipline and consistency are key with money.

So, are you good or bad with numbers? If you are good at

them, continue to apply this in your calculations, business and daily life. Everything is based on numbers, even going back thousands of years. Numbers have always been in existence to allow us to get through life, especially when it comes to money. Get clear with your numbers and always keep track of them.

How Much Would You Like to Earn?

Many times I have asked people, "How much money would you like to have" and they respond with . . . "As much as I can get!" or my favourite one "A million, if I were to win the lottery." These are ambitious goals, and are so vague to achieve success. It will be highly unlikely for the average person to achieve because most don't have a clear map or a wealthy income mindset. There are many wealthy people in this world who have not just become wealthy, through luck via a business or a highly paid job, they have developed a wealthy mindset which has attracted more wealth to them.

Is it possible for one person to be worth hundreds of thousands or millions? Of course. If they've worked hard, found a unique opportunity, and provided high value, then absolutely. Have you thought about how much you would like to earn? Never ever say it is impossible because there is always a way. You just have to go and seek it. There is a world of information out there that can help you do that. The likes of Warren Buffett, Bill Gates, Richard Branson and Jeff Bezos (founder of Amazon), who are the well-known self-made multi-billionaires of the world, have done just that.

My point, even they once started with perhaps just the amount of money that you have right now. So, what's the difference? They acted, they learned, they developed a wealthy mindset, they read books, they went to seminars, they made calls, they tried and failed. In the end, after all that, they then succeed. The key to earning more money is to just keep learning while you're earning.

Along the journey to increase your income, you may be faced with a few setbacks. However, if you keep going with determination and keep learning, I guarantee your income will increase. I gave up a highly paid job and my finances dwindled; then gradually over time, through continuously learning, consistency and persistence, I've managed to earn more and more, which will just continue to grow. Whenever I fail or lose, I park, I reflect and then I get back up again.

Richard Branson has stated, "Keep moving forward." "If a baby starts to walk and they fall; is the baby going to give up and just sit there for the rest of their life?" "No, they are going to get up and trying until they can walk." That's what you must do in life for the growth of your financial income. Just keep moving. Forget about what other people think or say to you. Remove the self-doubts that you may have. Just keep moving forward. That's it! Identify how much you would like to earn, set goals, keep learning and be consistent. Also, don't be afraid to set the bar high. I guarantee if you do this, at some point it will happen. You're going to grow older anyway, so you might as well keep trying in the time you have.

Ways to Earn More Money

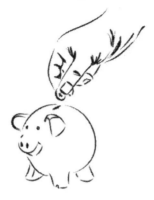

Today, the internet is the most advanced powerful driving force to deliver knowledge, communication, but most of all sales! Especially with the likes of Google, which have completely revolutionised and changed the world into a new age of information technology. Now, you can access a world of information almost anywhere at any point at any time.

There is just too much information right at your fingertips to not be able to leverage for a greater gain. I know of many successful online business owners, who have simply gone onto the Google search engine, typed in "how to make money" and then found a strategy and worked at it. Now, the strategy may have not created the success they wanted immediately, but they sought the information to find out where to start. Now, there are a few ways that you can make money online. Not all are easy by no means, particularly if you are not 'tech savvy.' I do have experience in digital marketing, does that make it easier for me to earn money online, probably. You need to have the right platform, system, training and product in place. By having these things in place, there are various ways that you can earn more money online. Keep reading, and all will be revealed.

To earn more money, the first thing you could do is perhaps look for a new job, which is fine. Alternatively, you could ask for a salary increase or promotion on your job. If you really like your job and would like more money but too afraid to ask, try to build up the courage and just ask your boss. The worst they can say is no, and if this is the case, you can consider one of two things:

1. You know where you stand to make the next decision.
2. You've achieved mass courage which is not easy. If it's a yes, then it is a bonus.

Another way of earning more money is to see how you can leverage your time. For example, if you're in a job full time, working Monday-Friday, you could utilise pockets of time to start an online business. Starting small, and building on an automated online system over time can produce an income which is making the most of your time, while you continue to work in your full-time job. If you own a business that requires physical or technical activity, then time is your biggest asset in sales, labour, marketing, accounting etc. By leveraging your time by hiring other people to work on the less relevant tasks, you will increase time for high productivity that will lead to generate more revenue and profits.

Robert Kiyosaki, entrepreneur and author of the book *Rich Dad Poor Dad*, said the key to wealth is to have multiple streams of income coming in per month, wherever those avenues of income are coming from. It is good to have multiple streams income that you can build into assets, rather than having to rely on just one. Another way to earn more money would be to perhaps sell items that you don't want on online market places, such as eBay or Amazon, or other online selling platforms. I'm sure there is someone out there who could benefit from your unwanted items. Rather than the items occupying space, why not make some money off them.

Another method of earning money is to create your own product or sell other peoples' products that are already on the market. Think about what products you are passionate about and find a way of creating them. It could be a physical product, a unique handmade product or even an information product (which are becoming increasingly popular in our information age). Once identified, these can also be sold on global online selling platforms, giving you great opportunities that your product can reach a large number of people, which as a result will generate more sales.

An increasingly popular way to earn money is to become an online affiliate. An affiliate is somebody who will market or recommend someone's product on their behalf, and in return, you earn a commission for every product/service that is sold. There are various marketing strategies you could use to market an affiliate product, such as social media, email marketing, PPC (pay-per-click), blogging or maybe through word of mouth. By doing some research into the affiliate company's programs, products, and consumer demand, you could find a unique position to be in to generate good commission. Simply type 'affiliate + (a product)' into a search engine and there will be a list of affiliate programs linked to that product. Alternatively, there are affiliate companies such as Clickbank, Amazon Associates, or eBay that have a bank of listed products waiting to be published to the mass market online.

An alternative way to earn an extra income which is now quite common is 'Network Marketing,' where you can start your own home business that has already been set up for you. Basically, it is a business in a box, along with methods behind an affiliate. All the products are there for you, along with the business system, marketing tools, website and commissions. You've just got to market those products in the preferred way that suits you, in order to generate sales and commission. There are many Network Marketing companies that offer great benefits, and the business model can be scaled over a period of time through time leverage and automation. It is a great way to develop a business mindset, as well as give you the drive and hunger to be an entrepreneur, learning through 'personal development'.

If you can get it right and scale the additional income streams, it could be life changing for you! Think about how you could perhaps earn more money and look into the options. Never just settle for less or sit there thinking "that's not going to happen to me" because you won't know unless you try. If you don't try, then nothing changes. A good friend of mine, Vishal Morjaria, once told me that the secret to wealth is having the ability to sell. He said, "If you don't know how to sell, then you will be broke; but if you learn how to make sales you will be wealthy."

Here is a list of additional income options to generate more money:

- Seek a higher paid job
- Ask for a promotion in your current job
- Sell your unwanted items (online or offline)
- Start a part time business (product or service)
- Create and sell your own products (offline or online: Amazon / eBay)
- Sell other people's products online (affiliate program)
- Leverage and 'buy time' in your business, by outsourcing work to freelancers

Talking Numbers

Numbers are everywhere, we use them for lots of things to allow us make numerous calculations and measurements, but how much attention do we pay to them in terms of communicating messages? This may sound strange if you're hearing this for the first time; however, you wouldn't believe how many numbers are trying to communicate with you on a daily basis. According to 'sacred numerology' there are numbers that have sequences, which translate into messages and meanings. Whether it is checking the clock for the time or checking how much is in your bank account, there are numbers that are constantly trying to give you a message that could well have some significance in your life at that present time.

In the spiritual realms of this world, there are numbers trying to tell you something which could either lead you to prosperity, steer you away from potential threats or towards the realisation of a life lesson. Have you ever looked at a digital clock and noticed any double numbers? You probably have, but never paid any attention to it. If you have noticed this or started to pick up on this, keep a very close eye if they continuously appear when you check the time. They are called 'angel numbers' which become more and more dominant day by day. For a deeper insight into this, run an internet search on 'Angel Numbers Index' to see what your numbers are trying to tell you. Once you do this, try to keep track of the numbers you repeatedly observe. Jot them down if you have to. This could be highly valuable to you. If you are an optimistic person, you are probably more likely to be able to open your mind a little further. Refer back to being a child again, think of how anything is possible because when you're a child, anything *is* possible. Your imagination was limitless, but as you grow up, you tend to lose that feeling of freedom in the mind. A great friend of mine, Wesley Bollington, founder of the 'Winkkey' app and expert in sacred geometry, can read persona types and significant events in someone's life, just by reading their numbers. Wow! The next time you see any numbers of significance, research into them and ask the question, "What are they trying to tell me?"

Money versus Time

Throughout the ages of time we have been constantly consumed and in some cases, controlled by money. It is what makes the world go around to an extent. People need to work at something to generate money. Businesses need to communicate with other businesses or consumers to make profit. We all need money to survive in some form or another! Zig Ziglar once said, "Money isn't everything, but it ranks right up there with oxygen." This is very true. We do need money in order to survive, but its not *everything*. The point I am trying to make is that you can always gain more money somehow; 'this is fantastic', unfortunately you can't retain more time. Once the day has passed, you can never get it back. You've probably heard the saying "You can't change the past, but you can change the future." Have a think about the amount of money you want to consume. Think about how you can invest your time for greater monetary gain for the future. Look at your outgoings versus your income and put it all into perspective.

To summarise this subject, your time is more valuable than money. You only have one life and there are only so many hours in a day, so choose how you spend it wisely. I tend not to waste my time in a day, not for anything nor anybody, because I understand how invaluable it is. Sometimes, I have to go out of my way and I have to use my time in terms of serving and helping others, which is what I love doing, but if I know that somebody or something is going to draw away my time that isn't worth my time, then it is a big fat **No**! The focus on my goals for income geared towards my vision is imperative to me.

Stephen Covey author of *The 7 Habits of Highly Effective People*, created a model in his book, which is the call the 'Time Management Quadrant.' There are four elements to this incredible model, each symbolising a different scenario, which will ultimately clarify the sufficiency of where your

time is best spent for maximum positive impact. *(I will discuss this in more detail in a later chapter).*
 Utilise your time wisely, and look at the bigger picture. Mind-sight over eye-sight.
 Remember these words... "You can get more money, but you cannot get more time."

Need some guidance on money management and income? visit www.changeitbook.com

Voices of 'Less' Value

I remember a time, during my twenties, when socialising with friends and family was the pinnacle point of my life. Together we had some memorable times and shared many ups and downs, which formed unbreakable bonds, that at a time I thought it would be endless. Until one day, I decided that I was going to take charge of my life, after detrimental events had taken place over a few years. I became tired of mediocrity, and wasn't going to settle for an average life by following the crowd. I was going to do something new for the better, something which was for me and only me. This was a revelation to me! However, unfortunately, not everyone in my immediate circle agreed with this new philosophy on life. There were those who disagreed with my new choices, some even thought I was crazy, they just couldn't understand or recognise what I was going through at that time.
 Most people don't like change, even when they will benefit so much more if they take the leap. It is not completely their

fault, it's our brain that puts up survival barriers to protect you from potential danger. The brain dislikes any type of unfamiliar habits or behaviours, hence the reason it can be extremely difficult for some people to embrace the thought of change. So, they will stay within their comfort zone, where the brain is telling them that they are safe. What they don't realise, is that the challenges on the outside of the comfort zone are where you eventually achieve the things that you desire most.

One day, I met up with a friend for a social catch up; although, I already knew that he didn't agree too much with my new ventures and philosophies of life. Around that time, I had started a new business (albeit very small) which was something fairly new to the market. I gained quite a few customers, and I started to make some steady progress. Previously, my friend and I could talk about life, women, work, the fun times, etc, which was great. However, when a business-related topic came up in conversion, I knew the conversation was going to turn into a different (and not so great) direction.

He asked how the new business venture was going and I replied; "Yes, it's steady, but going well." In my head, I knew where this was heading, so I attempted to change the subject. I followed by saying, "I'm feeling quite happy in what I'm doing, thanks; do you mind if we can change the subject please?" Without listening to a word I just said, my friend replied, "I don't think what you are doing is a good idea." (Even though I just requested to change the subject). I suddenly became frustrated inside. I kindly said, "I understand you feel that way; however, I am really happy in what I'm doing, and hopefully one day I'll become a successful entrepreneur and . . ." Before I could even finish the sentence, I was rudely interrupted - "You are NOT an entrepreneur, you are NOT an entrepreneur!" "This will never work for you!"

At the back of my mind, I became emotionally drained, humiliated and alienated. I felt anger. I felt pain. I felt frustration and most of all, I felt a great loss of connection with a friend.

I paused, turned to him and said, "This is the start of my new life." "This is my new venture." "It's is my dream to become successful and help a lot of people in the process." "This feels right for me." After speaking my mind, by this point, I thought there would have been some understanding or even the slightest piece of encouragement, but unfortunately there was not. My friend simply came back with "Well, I completely disagree, it's a bad idea." "Just stick with a job, you're much better off."

At that moment, I realised that I was just talking to a brick wall. He couldn't see the potential gain and positive impact it was having on my life. I suddenly realised that these brick walls would continue to be in the way of my goals, dreams and aspirations if I didn't make some changes with certain people. From that point on, my relationships with specific people who were in my life, were never the same. I began to identify the relationships and voices of those that were more toxic than empowering, which created distance. I then sought new friends through network events, workshops and social media who I attracted. They were genuine and more positive, that I could connect with and share good vibes and energies.

'Don't listen to the voices that don't count, seek the voices of good value.' - C.J. Alexander

Ever since that day, I have been extremely careful about who I spend my time with. It has been said that 'You become one of the five people that you spend the most time with.' Listen to the voices of those that count and have value, also those who will support you in your goals to create a better future.

You can't change people, people can only change themselves! I've learned this philosophy over the last few years, and due to this slight shift in thinking, I now have good close friends. I limit my time with certain family members and I spend more time with positive entrepreneurial friends who continue to inspire and motivate me.

STEP 5

Grow:
With or Without Others

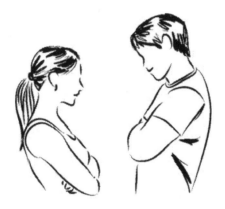

What Are You Absorbing?

Throughout each day, we are exposed to thousands of marketing messages and voices, which we consume. Most people are unaware of how these messages can have a significant impact on their life. This is the power of influence that is feeding your mind every day, year after year. Just take a minute and ask yourself these questions; What do I listen to? Who do I watch? What do I read? How do I act and behave to different people? Who do I spend most of my time with?

If you have answered the above questions honestly, the answers will determine the type of person that you are. Within minutes of having this conversation with yourself, you can identify why your life is like this and perhaps where it is heading. You've got to think outside of the box and look at your life from an outside perspective, rather than just what is in front of you. This will allow you to reveal some truths, correct the errors of the past and begin the new process of selective listening, in order to find the voices of value.

If your mind absorbs what is in the media such as the news and information surrounding all the negative impacts of the world, then what impact is this having on your thoughts and attitude? If you are a fan of the media because it is helping you in some way, that is absolutely fine, if that's what really makes you happy, for example, entertainment, sport or lifestyle etc. Just be wary of becoming too consumed by it in the long term, as the messages behind marketing brands can leave you with a dent in your wallet. If you really want to move forward with your life, then it might be a better idea to sketch out (on paper) the things you should be doing to feed your mind positively.

If you're a person like me, who continues to strive for more, and who is tired of settling for less, then collect a few books that have good value, read them and take some steps of action. Search and read articles online, seek advice from experts in a particular field, sign up to their newsletters, whatever it takes to constantly feed your mind, so that it is filled with clear nourishing knowledge rather than unhealthy toxic junk. Most people will say to themselves, "I haven't got the time, I'm just too busy to focus on anything else." Well, if you can't make the time right now, don't stress yourself out about it, just allocate some dedicated time when you can, and be consistent with your new schedule. Let me give you a scenario as an example of how two people with the same time constraints end up with different outcomes. Both people want to lose weight of 15 pounds. Person A decides to eat an apple every day for a full 365 days. Then cuts out chocolate, junk foods and lower their carb intake. Person B decides to try a similar diet while watching food shows, and occasionally visit fast food stores. At the end of the first month, the Person B says, "You know what, this diet is not really for me. I will cut out the other stuff, but I will keep eating chocolate." Then they carry on doing that for the remaining part of the year. At the end of the year, Person A achieves the goal of losing 15 pounds; however, Person B ends up gaining an additional 10 pounds. Two people had the same goal and the same length of time, but slightly different attitudes, which produced different results. What was the difference??? 1. Their attitude, 2. Their actions. My point is, when you feed your mind, it permits focus, which develops into progress, but if it is not consistent you will keep stopping and starting, ending up either back to square one or in a worse situation than when you began.

Take some time out to really think about the voices and messages that you are feeding your mind. What are you feeding your mind daily? What are you listening to daily? What do you read daily? What are you continuously absorbing in your environment? These factors will determine the type of person you will become. What would you rather do? Fill your glass up with dirty water? Or fill your glass with pure, crystal clear water, so that you have more control over your life with a clear vision.

Who Are You Around?

This is by far one the most crucial fundamentals of this chapter, if not of the book. It is imperative to identify the people that you are around and who you are spending most of your time with. They say that you become one of the five people that you're around most. This isn't an assumption; it is a fact! Believe it or not, this philosophy does impact people throughout their lives. Yet, most are still oblivious to this concept, and wonder why their lives have turned out that way. The people we are around most, are a massive influence in our lives, from the things they say, their behaviours and actions, all impact our lives, and subsequently our own thoughts and actions. Why try to fit in, when you were born to stand out!

Think about all the things people do and say that dictate the way you feel. If you are very independent and driven by your own motives, and don't care about what other people think, then good for you! We tend to lean towards what others think a lot of the time, which unfortunately often dictate our actions in life. We listen to what other people think, and we take it onboard if we feel it is of value. If someone criticises or belittles us, some may believe that it is true, especially if the judgement was made by someone who is close to them, but it is not always true. It's only true if you say it is. That's why it is important to have a positive and bold frame of mind in order to raise your self-esteem and build on your confidence. Please, know that this is your life, and you deserve to live it the way you wish.

Ask yourself this . . . "With these people around me, what am I becoming? What have they got me saying and believing? How have they influenced me to act?" These are all factors that will dictate your life. If there is a part of your life that you're not happy with, and that includes certain people who you are around; then, you must make some serious changes. Family is always a tricky one, so if possible, create some space and reduce time spent with them, if they are holding you back. If they are friends or associates, then start moving into new circles. People will try and dictate to you on how you should live your life, but is it what you truly want? It is okay to make changes, so don't be afraid, and it is okay to move on and leave people behind. At the end of the day, YOU can only live your life. No one else can.

The Power of Influence

The power of influence is all the influence of those who we choose to listen to, and those around us (as previously mentioned in this chapter). From the people that we're around, to what we're listening to and what we're reading and absorbing on a daily basis, each hour, day, week, month, year etc. 99% of influences will dictate the person that we have become. If you break it down into certain segments to identify who or what is causing your manifestation of character, it will determine the power of the influence for the future. For many years I've listened to a lot of people assuming that what I was hearing was wisdom for a great future. I thought this was great and classified myself very lucky. I have been really successful in my education, my career, my personal and professional friendships, but then, only a few years ago, I had a light bulb moment when a friend wasn't so supportive in my decisions and actions of pursuing. That person tried to persuade me into doing something else, which I knew deep down wasn't right for me.

The reality is that many people go through life saying 'Yes' because it is easier, but sometimes you have to say No. If you don't say no, then you end up being led down a path which you could later regret. We should be able to say what's in our heart and what is backed up by our instinct, but due to peer pressure and the fear of being judged, we often go with the opposite. What matters is how you feel within yourself, your heart and your gut. Be aware of the power of influence, be strong and be bold to stand up for what is right for you.

Time to Grow

After reading the previous few chapters of this book, you're probably starting to build an understanding of the important elements to consider when making changes in your life. It all starts with your 'philosophy' and way of thinking to develop a unique mindset, to be able to grow within yourself and make better decisions with your health, relationships and income. Think about some of the things that we've discussed, such as how your health should be and what you 'should' / 'should not' be putting into your body. What goals you should set, how to dream big and what you would like to aspire for. Keeping track of the numbers for financial gain, and how numbers can serve you for a great purpose. By combining all these, you should begin a process of ideas and new undiscovered concepts that will enable you to move forward for a better future.

Growing is such a great thing, it does something to feed the mind and the soul. However, like a flower, if you're not growing, then you're dying. We can either learn to adapt and grow to move forward or take no new action and be held back. Other people's influences can play a part in resistance to change, but the other part is to do with our self-doubt, leading with our head rather than our heart. It can paralyse us from doing great things if we don't take those small action steps. There is always something inside that holds us back, and with the oppression of self-doubt holding you back, it won't allow you to grow if you don't step into your fears. If you say "I can" rather than saying, "I can't" it is more likely to empower you the more you say it.

Due to the complexities of life, in whatever situation we are in, excuses will always be at the forefront before action is taken to develop and facilitate self-growth. If you say "I can do this, because I must do this" it will start to build that small spark of courage and confidence in yourself. When you do eventually take action, and begin to grow by investing in yourself, you will sooner or later bloom like a beautiful flower above the rest.

Growing is part of a 'doing' process, but more importantly part of a 'becoming' process. The greatest things in life are not what you do or what you possess; the greatest thing is what you become! 80% Growing 20% Doing. Substantial growth comes from learning. If you wish to grow, the answers are in books! Become an excellent reader, and an excellent listener. With the advance of technology in the 21st century, such as podcasts and the increasingly popular online phenomenon YouTube, watching and listening to online videos is one of the fastest ways to learn. In my eyes, one of the most powerful ways to learn and build new philosophies is to go to live events.

Events have been my secret source of building upon success in self-development and in business. There is something special about attending an event that will enable self-belief, new confidence, and the courage to break out of your comfort zones. Build upon new conversations with like-minded people and you can stretch your thinking rather than being stuck around those who are hopelessly lost, who will only hold you back.

It is very difficult to transform your current state overnight into an alter ego of incredible inner power and substantial self-growth; this takes time. Growth and success will occur by learning, not only in the gathering of new knowledge, but also in the development of new emotions through experiences. As you gradually keep growing and building new connections, you will continue to grow into the person that you could have only imagined.

Attitude

What shapes our attitude? I guess most of the time it is down to our beliefs, but the power of influence plays a huge role. It's what we know and what we feel that determines our attitude. We must make sure that our emotions are in check. Sometimes, we will hear things and say things, and how we react to these will determine our attitude. Daily habits that are picked up can also shape our attitude.

Some people have their emotions intact, but this is rare and can be difficult to master. If others say certain things to them, they will not allow the emotional side to get the best of them, instead they react to the comment in a calm way. However, others who are not so skilled in mastering the control of their emotions don't tend to think, and can become verbally reactive in a not so pleasant way.

It's okay to kick and scream when you are the age of three, but not when you are thirty-three. Having your emotions intact can benefit you greatly, so that you can deal with situations appropriately rather than flying off the handle, which can allow people to humiliate themselves and look unprofessional, especially within a workplace.

Have you ever come across those people that you said the wrong words to, and they erupted like a volcano? They're the ones I am talking about.

On the other end of the spectrum, you have people who will take criticism and won't say anything back. In some cases, it is nice to keep the peace, but that can become damaging to your self-esteem in the long run. There must be a balance between the two. If you want to shape your attitude for positive gain, and you're around people who are not doing you any good, then don't talk like they talk or walk like they walk. Don't listen to what they are listening to. Don't act like they do. Develop new behaviours and habits that you can build daily to shape your attitude.

Emotions can either embarrass you or support you. One way of mastering this is to find an expert, or someone who you highly value, who you want to aspire to be like. Attitude is such a powerful thing to have, because it can determine the path that you take in life. It can determine your choices and develop confidence for you to express your values, rather than hesitate and hold you back. Every choice that we make based on our attitude can shape our destiny. I believe one of the most important aspects of an attitude is our self-worth. The more self-worth we retain, the more we will increase the good feelings and attitude toward ourselves and others.

There are three main elements of attitude; what we know, how we feel, and what we do. These three elements, combined with self-worth, make it possible to make a paradigm shift in thinking to be able to walk out of the darkness into the light. It will enable you to come from a place of heartbreak into unbelievable self-confidence, leading to self-transformation.

Love

There are numerous people that we come into contact with throughout our lives, some who are with us for most of it, then some who come and go. Love, however, is the most powerful force of nature in this world. From the minute we were born, we know in our hearts that we are meant to love. We know the things that we love, and we know the things that we don't, by the way we feel. Whether it is your partner, family or friends that you are with, the power of love will always draw you to that person. Love is truth. 'Love your neighbour as yourself.' *Galatians 5:14. N.I.V*

We touched on this subject in a previous section, about those who we want to be around and those people who we don't. In order to grow, we sometimes need to make difficult choices and let some people go to live their path. But we must try to maintain positive or civil relationships with our close loved ones. You might not always see eye to eye with what you're trying to achieve (especially if it is concerning making changes to your life), but you can still love them for who they are. As well as following a path that your heart is telling you to, it can be difficult to have others understand your point of view. They love you, and they just don't want you to get hurt as a result of the change. If you communicate with them on their level, let them know, that whatever worries or concerns they have, you value their concerns very much. Let them know, this is something that you wish to do because it is in your heart to do it. Don't feel that you need to change your new found attitude, by allowing others to tripwire you through criticism or guilt. This reaction is often down to their own fears about making changes in their own life, and how risk averse they are.

Find the love for what you want to do, love to fulfil your purpose, and love for that person that you sincerely want in your life. It is important to love the ones that are dear to us, as it is important to love ourselves. More importantly, it is imperative to be in love with what you do in life. If you can find passion and love for what it is that you really want to do, I guarantee your life will become full of abundance and prosperity. Seek love in all things and follow your heart.

Your Inner Power

You have the ability in this world to do anything that you feel can be achieved. What have you achieved so far, that at the start, you thought you couldn't? Those were things that you thought were near impossible, but you managed to get from A to B, whether it was a task, assignment, project, new job or business venture. If this is you, I want to congratulate you for tapping into your inner power and cutting through the challenges. I'm sure you've heard of the saying, "If you put your mind to it, you can do it;" that it is possible for most things that you really want to achieve in life.

I'm sure, many times, you may have doubted yourself by thinking, "I don't know how I'm going to be able to achieve this," then the self-doubt starts to creep in and paralyse you. Saying "I can" rather than, "I can't" can develop your attitude and develop that feeling of excitement to forge ahead and pursue your goals. Keeping people around us who bring us down and bring negativity into our lives, can suppress our inner power. Creating space for yourself from the 'psychic vampires' that try to suck the life out of your inner power will allow the time to develop your attitude and confidence to achieve great things.

This growing self-confidence, faith in yourself and the spirit (if you feel connected with spirituality) helps to unfold the hidden power. It is known that there are powers and principalities of this world that we don't even know exist, because they're not seen or heard. They are there to fuel us in times of need, to reveal the depths of inner strength both physically and mentally. There is an inner power of greatness in you to shape your destiny.

For more advice on self-development to grow
abundantly, visit www.changeitbook.com

STEP 6

Excitement:
Be Excited about
Your Future

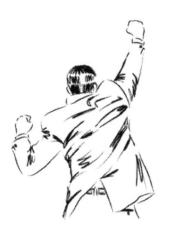

Get Excited!

I revealed in chapter three, how to aspire for more, so that you can set your goals, paint the vision of where you would like to be, and then work towards the fulfilment of these goals. Once you have built a vision in your mind and gained a sense of exhilaration, you must keep hold of that feeling, treasure it and protect it! Most days I used to wake up and open the window and just look out onto the water. I would drift off into a daydream (just for a couple of minutes), of what my life would be like, having achieved different elements of the incredible vision. It created that little buzz which expanded into a stronger feeling of excitement. There's nothing better than the feeling of EXCITEMENT! It brings happiness. It brings joy. It brings butterflies of prosperity geared towards what is to come.

Being excited will bring hope and will continue to allow you to grow, but there is a catch to this feeling. Life can often get in the way of your pleasant moments and if you allow it, it can zap those most precious feelings of abundance. Please, don't lose sight of the vision, even when times feel hard or things might not go your way. When life knocks you down, gradually work your way back up to reach your place of peace. Try anything that makes you happy to give off a little bit of buzz of excitement.

What works for me, is to *listen to uplifting music,* watch TV shows or movies that make me laugh, spend time with friends, but most of all spending time with my daughter. Those little things can initiate feelings of happiness and excitement. As we grow older, we can be so consumed by life that we can forget the feelings that allow us to bloom; so get excited today about where your future is heading and where the vision will take you.

The Buzz Factor

Do you ever get that feeling sometimes deep down, that you're destined for great things? That you're put on this earth for a purpose? Let that be your inspiration to serve others; perhaps, even help hundreds, thousands, or maybe even millions of people. That is what creates a buzz factor, knowing that you have a purpose, knowing that you have a destiny to fulfil. With that exhilarating thought process, you can achieve extreme levels of excitement and overwhelming feelings of where your future is heading and where you want to arrive. This is all part of painting a vision and building the buzz factor, especially if you are someone who wishes to make a difference in the world.

My mantra is "I wish to travel the world, support and help others, and earn a good living from it." I use this every day to kick-start my buzz factor. I do this every single day (even at difficult times) to make sure that I'm keeping a small spark of excitement and ongoing self-belief. I have unlimited faith in God and myself that one day, it will manifest into full creation. I am familiar with various world-famous individuals who are known for such works in affirmations. Tycoons for example are, John Asaraf, Tony Robbins, Darren Hardy and many more who have impacted thousands of lives just by teaching simple yet incredible strategies to unleash strong affirmations that are then embedded in their minds. This will build upon the buzz factor to enable the change. These experts never stopped working on this until they achieved their goals. Today, they have helped thousands upon thousands of people to achieve goals and change their lives. Pretty awesome right?

Find something that makes you happy or a passion, to create a vision. Find ways of making a change, whether it be with your health, relationships or income, and keep working on the buzz factor for sparks of excitement.

What Creates Excitement?

Often, we get excited about various things, which might be as simple as coming home to see your loved ones, children, partner, or your pet. It could be another form of excitement, for example; when you know you're going to purchase something you can't wait to receive, and you know it is coming, or when you have booked a vacation and you just can't wait to get away because you know you have worked so hard for the break.

However, sometimes, excitement can come from within. It can occur regardless of where you are or what situation you're in. Be in tune with finding something that you can work towards that's going to give you excitement. You don't necessarily need materialistic items to give you excitement. You can be excited right now, today, if you paint the vision big enough of where you want to go and the person you want to become. That's what excites me the most! We go through different stages throughout every year and some things are really exciting for us, some things we just want to avoid. At times, it can be quite hard for us, because life is hard and can draw you towards pain. Les Brown said in one of his great motivational speeches, "In life, there's too much pain to duck. It's everywhere! At some point, it will come and find you." We must rise above it when we can, by summoning the strength to move forward and keep focused on the excitement of our goals.

Once you decide on what you want your health to be like, what you want your relationships to be like (whether it is personal, professional or social) and the type of income you want to earn, you can produce indestructible confidence and self-belief based on the possibilities and excitement that you can create.

Having It and Keeping It

Your self-belief will keep you going in terms of how much your excitement is going to stay with you. I've had many visions of where my life is going to lead, which the average person would probably think "Oh, well, it's just a dream. That will never happen to me."

The one thing I can say, is that I have researched many successful people around the world who have achieved fulfilment in their lives based on the principles discussed in this chapter. I read a book once called *Beach Money* by Jordan Adler. In his book, he tells the story of how he spent over 10 years searching for an opportunity that could not only work for him but ultimately change his life. He said that he had nothing at one point, all he did was work full time at a job for not much in return, but he always had a hunger to strive for more. Then one day, he stumbled across a book for 25¢ that he could learn from to perhaps make some changes to his life.

After reading this book, he went for a quiet walk in the forest; a place of peace and tranquillity. He took out a journal, a pen and began to scribe his dream life, exactly the way he wanted it to be, including all the details of how it would look and how it would feel. He continued to do that for a number of years and would read his notes over and over again, feeding his mind with visions, hope and faith, until one day he decided to put it away and continue with his journey.

Years later, he had finally achieved success and managed to transform his life. He found all the things that he had wanted: a beautiful home, all the income that he dreamt about, the support of his family and friends, and the positive relationships that had developed over the years. One day, while sorting through some stuff he came across that same old journal he first started to write in about his dream life. After sitting down and flicking through the pages, he couldn't believe that all the things that he had wanted had manifested into his dream life, near enough word for word. Wow! Now here is the interesting part. If he hadn't started writing in his journal there probably is a great possibility that he may not have achieved what he had set out to. Writing in his journal had great significance in developing a strong subconsciousness, along with the tenacity to work hard for this magnificent life transformation.

I'm no psychic, but what I do know is that putting those words onto paper, having never ending self-belief, faith and the inclination to work hard, was a significant contributing factor to manifest his perfect life. This is all down to belief in knowing that you can achieve the things you want, to manifest your desires into creation. If that doesn't excite you, and start to get the blood pumping, then I don't know what will.

Remember, at the same time you can be happy, and you can be excited just by focusing on a brighter future, despite what others might say or think; that's their business, not yours; so, don't allow anyone to dull your sparkle of excitement. Just focus on you and where your excitement is going to take you. Hold on to it, treasure it and protect it.

The Law of Attraction

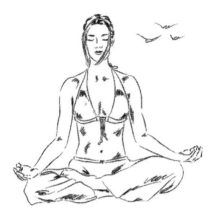

If you haven't heard of this concept, then you will be blown away by this (that is if you are an optimist). The law of attraction is a philosophy that can 'attract' things into your life, regardless of whether it is positive or negative. It is the manifestation of thoughts that turn into reality. Ask, Believe, and Receive.

Our thoughts are made up of energy. When we use the law of attraction, that energy attracts a 'like' energy, which can have a huge impact on our health, relationships and income. I first discovered this concept for myself when I watched the movie *The Secret, but the concept is as old as the universe with its principles firmly based on quantum physics.* The philosophy behind it is that your thoughts become things within reality. Have you ever felt that some aspects of your life have somehow fallen into place? Or you have negative areas in your life which keep appearing and just keep spiralling out of control? It took me years of wondering, why certain things turned out the way they did in life. Most of the time, it is our subconscious mind that is in fact creating those thoughts, which begin to manifest into reality. Whatever I focused on most and thought about was forming into energies and beliefs, which was attracting more of it in my reality, whether positive or negative. The problem with the 'Law of Attraction' is that it doesn't know the difference between positive or negative, so be careful of what you ask for.

Taking a step back from reality and thinking about the things that we really want can create positive energies, but also, be good for the mind to give you hope and excitement. It can feed your desires and eliminate the fears, block out all the rubbish that's going on around you. Slowly but surely, when you build in the habit of 'thought focus' you will start to attract more of it.

Now beware, things do not appear the next day like you have a genie in a lamp, asking for desires on demand. This is not how it works! It involves focus, time and most of all work. As Jim Carrey said on a show with Oprah "You can't ask for what you want and then go get an ice cream, it involves hard work." If you wish to be a millionaire tomorrow and you are broke, it is highly unlikely to happen. But if you set some goals, create a plan, use the concept of the law of attraction, with hard work, then it may just work for you in time. Start by thinking of the small things that you want to come into your life which will make you a little bit happier and bring joy into your life.

Build this into a daily habit and you will start to see the Law of Attraction working for you. Remember, thoughts become things. Just think about something that gives you a sense of joy and continue to work on that.

Do not neglect this practice if you are not seeing results straight away. It takes focus, time and work! Remember, the law of attraction does not know the difference between positive and negative. Be conscious. If you ask and believe, you can receive and achieve.

Destiny Tuning

Like the Law of Attraction, we must ask, believe and then 'wait' until we receive, in order for the universe to put into place the things we desire. But there's a deeper methodology behind the 'Law of Attraction' that can make your desire become more of a reality with a much faster concept called 'Destiny Tuning.'

Destiny tuning is an approach to take control of your future effectively, so that it can manifest into what you want in your life. It is a proven scientific success principle for exceptionally focused minds, so that they can hit the bull's eye of their desires and allow them to manifest into reality. Call it an advanced level of the Law of Attraction.

The difference between destiny tuning compared to the Law of Attraction is that, it has more of a systematic appr-oach , following a step- by-step guide to allow manifest-ations of what you desire to take place, whereas, the Law of Attraction is a case of asking, believing and then assuming that you will receive what you want.

With destiny tuning, the mind becomes a focus point and connects with vibrations that ascend to new levels of abundance; in other words, using strong concentration levels, meditation and focus on desires, built upon more and more each day. It takes practice, focus and guarding against other thoughts and voices. Thoughts must be used to their full potential to create abundance. Attention to detail, including visions, environment, feelings, even smell and taste will work on your belief systems to manifest the desire into certainty.

The human mind is capable of multiplying its vibration frequency levels to match your individual desires. The more you are in tune with your destiny tuning, the more likely you are to manifest your desires into your destiny. If you believe this could work for you, try it for yourself and get in tune with your desires by just spending a few minutes each day in pure, concentrated meditation in a quiet place. Do it with joy and an open mind. If you are someone who is spiritual, this is probably going to work a lot faster than someone who perhaps isn't. If you do try this and become heavily in tune with your destiny, there is no doubt you will see a positive change in your life.

Your Future Awaits

When you have set your mind to have a crystal-clear vision of what your life will be like, all the things you will have, the people that will be a part of it, the things you will experience and the feeling of ultimate gratitude, is it all there waiting for you in the future. Isn't that exciting? It is possible to achieve your dreams and desires, whatever they may be. You can achieve them one by one, if you truly believe you will. The manifestation of each goal and desire will eventually come true. The key to this is to keep it stored as your hidden treasure at the back of your sub-conscious mind. You may have created a vision board of a collage of images and keywords for the desires. If so, use this as an amplifier to bring the desires to the forefront of your mind for a boost in focus.

By having this located in a familiar place to view daily, you can trigger blissful thought processes of the desires. Many people do this and guess what? It works! For some, desires will manifest, for others there won't. Why? . . . lack of focus, patience and hard work. NEVER give up your belief or hope. It is important to be excited as often as you can, knowing in faith that you will make it. Have you heard the saying "just three feet from gold?" You could be virtually at the tipping point of achievement, so don't give up. The second you turn away and give up on those goals and desires, it could be all lost.

The point I'm making here is that the time is going to pass anyway; so, you might as well make good use of it to build your future. Keep hold of that feeling of excitement and do not neglect it. Use this as an inspiration and motivation to keep you going, especially in times of self-doubt, knowing it is possible for you. No matter how big or small or what anybody else says to you, these are your goals and dreams NOT theirs. Keep focused, view your vision board regularly and keep working towards your goals and dreams with excitement. Your future awaits!

Want to master the art of building excitement? visit www.changeitbook.com

STEP 7

Implementation: Take Action Now

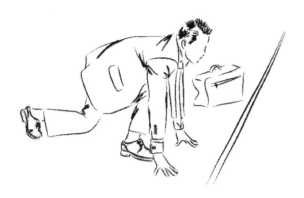

Learn and Execute

Over the last few years, I have read countless books; approximately one book a month on various topics including health, personal development, philosophy, business, marketing, money, spirituality, relationships and communication. Accumulating different pieces of knowledge has continuously built the foundations, which then became embedded in my mind as a source of a new philosophy. This has made magnificent changes in my life, which is why I am sharing this knowledge with you.

Many of these teachings came from experts in different fields and have been developed from my own personal experiences. This will forever continue to develop the more I learn in terms of knowledge, but more importantly within myself. The point I'm making is that you have got to keep learning and working on yourself by taking action. If you have a hunger for learning to achieve more and fulfil your true potential, then keep going! Like the saying in business, the more you learn, the more you earn.

On top of the learning, it is about taking action and execution. What you are learning? How much action are you taking based on the teachings? Without implementation, you will just end up at the same spot. If this type of behaviour is repeated, this is how we become stuck. If you find any piece of information relevant to you, put it into practice, even if it is only a small step toward the change. Whether this is regarding your health, relationships, or income, you must implement action along with knowledge building, in order to solidify the change. That way, you will learn, stretch yourself and begin to put the wheels of manifestation into motion. Learn as much as you can, and don't stop. You're either growing or you're dying. Be specific in what you want, and learn on how you can achieve it with action whenever you can. Wealthy people have a habit of getting things done much faster than most (yes, they may have the financial backing, but they tend to move quickly). This creates momentum, thus more success is achieved. However, this is not just for money and wealth, this is about all applying these principles to all the areas of your life that need attention. Just keep building upon the knowledge, act with intent, and be consistent.

Why Implementation?

Can we make improvements by doing nothing? The answer is absolutely no! Most people want to move forward, get off the mark, make and allow some transformation in their lives. The problem is that they do nothing, wish and wait for things to happen. Some people get fired up and say "Yeah, I'm going to use the law of attraction. I just know it's going to happen for me," but then do nothing. It doesn't work without implementation. Some type of physical activities must take place, that may well be out of your comfort zone, in order for you to move forward.

It is often said that "we struggle to make change, because we fear the change in itself" but it is essential to keep on doing the work in order to create improvement. You may want to take some actions for better health, to lose weight or increase fitness, a change in mindset to reduce daily stress or take time out to recharge your exhausted body. If the change you want is related to a relationship issue, then you may want to take the relationship to the next level by confronting the other person and telling them how you feel; not always the easiest of tasks, I know. It may be to change something in your career, job or business. If you really want to allow some form of transformation, taking the leap to make that change will help you massively. You will achieve so much from taking the leap. Nine times out of ten, it is the fear that holds us back from taking that initial leap.

We get so confused sometimes about what to do; we get caught up with conflict in the mind which can create anxiety and stress, not knowing where to turn. A confused mind doesn't really do anything, it just stays where it is, going back and forth with repeated thoughts, but a focused and strategic mind will move you forward. If there's anything I have learned from my experiences, it is to make plans, and put them into action.

Step by step, jumping through a few hoops, will allow change to take place. As I mentioned earlier, taking small steps is worth a hundred years of thinking about it. One hundred years of thinking??? No Thanks! Just by taking that one first step, regardless of how scary it may be, at least you can say, "I did it. I tried it, I took action and moved slightly towards the goal." That is how important implementation is, and we must take full advantage of this concept in the areas of our lives, when we wish to improve.

Procrastination versus SOI (Speed of Implementation)

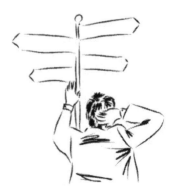

To get through life, we have to get things done. There is no way around it except for taking action. If you want to move forward, sitting around and wishing for things to happen is not going to work. It is so easy to want to do something, but the work that comes with it can lead to procrastination to set in. Delaying things by putting them off just defeats the objectives. Accomplishing even one task is a step toward completion, rather than nothing at all. If you take one step a day or one step a week towards a goal, it can make all the difference. The quicker you take more steps, then the quicker you will accomplish your goals, but it has got to be CONSISTENT, which will then lead to significant progress. Consistency never fails, but contemplating can steer you off track.

Goals are important! Dreams are important! But the action is even more crucial. The 'baby steps' to getting to where you want to be will eventually turn into larger accomplishments in your health, income and relationships, which will take them to the next level. It is known that we tend to procrastinate, depending on how undisciplined we are. Students who attend college or university will often procrastinate until the last minute of an assignment's deadline. Why is this common among students? It is because of the lack of pressure and consequence; we know that we have to get things done, but we assume at first that we have time to waste before we take action. We wait and keep putting it off until the pressure kicks in, then have grave penalties to face. If you are able to overcome the procrastination and just 'do something,' this will work better for you in the long run.

It is like being in a car and setting the destination in the navigation system, to go from place A to place B. You can't move anywhere unless you turn on the ignition in the car.

It is as simple as that. Turning on the ignition is the first step, followed by acceleration, gears, etc. Now, it might not feel like you are getting anywhere near the destination or goal at first, but once the car starts to roll and the wheels start to turn, you begin moving forward making steady progress. As you are travelling, you will pick up speed and there will be times that you slow down, but with consistency and the increase in speed, you will eventually get there. It is the speed of implementation (SOI) that makes a difference in how fast you get things done. As my online mentor, Tai Lopez, would say "You've just got to get things done!" I myself, after many years of teaching students, had to constantly and consistently adapt to change and move forward. If I had not taken this approach and had instead chosen paths of procrastination, then, all hell would have broken loose during the stages of my teaching career, and I would have become unsuccessful.

Do you want to be someone who moves slowly forward? Or stay in your comfort zone, not doing much and procrastinating? Or choose the SOI path and move FASTER? Become the one who gets things done and allows change to form in your life, by implementing steps and applying speed.

Mindset Shift

This is the start, the omega, the 'be all' of your attitude towards things that you do in your life; it all starts in the mind. Our mindset controls our emotions, our attitude and our strength, both mental and physical. Whatever we ask for and believe in, we can achieve. This comes from the mind. Having a well-structured and focused mindset can determine the path that you will lead.

If your mindset is weakened by self-doubt, anxiety, depression or stress, this can ultimately distract you from where you would want to be in your life. If you are a person who tends to beat themselves up, complain and say "why hasn't it happened for me yet?" there will be blocks in your progress until you release those negative energies, by paying no attention to them.

You can develop a great mindset by learning from those who have good mindsets. Look at their attitudes, their behaviours, their habits and their use of vocabulary. All these qualities are signs of positive vibes, depending on what type of mindset you wish to grow.

A number of times, I have heard people say, "If you want success or change, it's about changing your mindset." I used to get so frustrated by this statement because it sounded so easy coming from others, yet it was so difficult for me to make that immediate shift. So, I had to ask myself 'What type of mindset do I want?' then I began to search for the ideal mentor who I could learn to develop the shift in mindset. You can seek it either by finding someone with a good mindset or doing the research into the skills. If you are like me who loves to learn, then perhaps do both. The greatest way is to replicate those with a bold and *optimistic* mindset. It is the same with your relationships, if you would like more connection, communication or intimacy, then an expert or coach on these areas will help you to make that shift.

My question to you is; what type of mindset do you

want to have? Also, do you know anyone with a mindset you would like to have? If you do, then perhaps ask them a few questions about how they work on their mindset and what skills they have acquired. It might well be a simple set of principles that make the difference. Just by asking them what gets their mindset in gear, could be a game changer for you.

This subject relates to chapter five of this book, where I talked about being on the right path and who you are with along that path. You will become one of the five people that you spend most of your time with. Whatever energies their mindset is giving off (attitude, behaviours and habits) you will have the tendency to draw towards it, feed off it and eventually replicate it. Having your own focused and independent mindset is an incredible attribute to have. It is okay to be different. Why try to fit in, when you were born to Stand Out! Don't let those people keep nudging you, feeding you comments, telling you what to do or allowing their opinions to affect you. This starts out as a slight elbow in your back and before you know it, you are off track of your goals and dreams completely. Be very wary of what you are absorbing in your mind and how your mindset is developing. Guard and protect it!

Consistency

Consistency is one of the most powerful disciplines you can have in order to succeed in anything. Look at some of the world's sporting greats who are phenomenal achievers such as Michael Jordan in basketball, Tiger Woods in golf, Serena Williams in tennis, Cristiano Ronaldo in football,

Lewis Hamilton in the Formula 1 and Floyd Mayweather in boxing.

These are all highly-skilled masters in their sporting fields. They say it takes an average of 10,000 hours to become a master at something. This mastery obviously does not happen overnight. To master anything, you must be consistent with focus, have an unbreakable bond of passion and work your damn ass off! That is why all the celebrity sport individuals have really become so great at their sport. They mastered the game and mastered their minds. They ate, slept and dreamt about their sport, along with years of discipline and time investment, they are the ones who have stood out in the world as the greatest.

What would you like to become really good at? Don't think for even a second that you can't achieve it, as this will place a block in your belief system. Think about what it is that you could do, which is measurable and realistic with time invested to become a master. Just pick one thing and one thing only, don't be the jack of all trades and master of none. What can you master? Once you do become a master at it, you become an expert. Once you become an expert, people see you as an authority. When you become an authority, there is a good chance you can become really successful in the eyes of others. Then, when people know you as an authority combined with your success, you then become a celebrity in your own field. When you become a celebrity, there will be a lot of people who know you for your expertise in your mastered field. Then guess what happens . . . they will pay you big money to witness your mastery. Consistency leads to mastery!

What Can You Achieve?

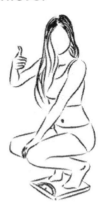

I've talked about ways to achieve your desires and there's no reason whatsoever why you can't aspire to achieve these things. For the next few minutes, I want you to think about the answers to the following questions. At this present time, what can you achieve? What skills do you have that can help you achieve a goal? We've previously established the significance of baby steps, and how its implementation can turn into great progress. So, what small steps can you take to achieve a goal for the first check point? By setting small check points towards your overall goals, you will be able to break up the overwhelming feelings, and give you faith in progress once each checkpoint is accomplished. It will increase motivation and recognition for unknown capabilities. The more you build up your recognition of each goal achieved, the more likely this will continue to expand into bigger and better things to take you to new heights.

If it is an income goal, how much do you want to achieve per month or per year? Whatever it is, break it down; so that the achievement becomes more realistic in a reasonable timeframe. Let's say in the next 12 months you want to achieve your ideal body weight or body shape by losing 30 pounds.

You could measure the progress of achievement like this:
30 pounds - divided by 12 months = 2.5 pounds per month

Or:

30 pounds - divided by 4 = 7.5 pounds every 3 months

Whatever type of goal you set, breaking it down into measurable check points will help massively. Whether it be a language or skill that you want to develop, or qualities in your personal or professional relationships, work with goal setting, action taking, consistency and measuring the progress.

What can you work on right now that's going to better yourself and help you grow? Think about some of the things you want to achieve, and work on the small steps because the more achievements you reach, the greater you will become. There's nothing better than the feeling of increasing your self-esteem and confidence by achievement.

Never Give Up: Just Keep Trying

When things that we want to achieve in life become overwhelming or challenging, it sometimes feels easier to just give up and say, "That's it! I have tried, I'm not getting anywhere, it is time to give up. I QUIT!" In most cases, that's what people do. They tend to just give up rather than pursue the goal and just keep going that little bit further until they reach the tipping point of success.

Yes, of course, like most, I have given up on things before too; that's part of life. But when your sole mission, purpose and desire is to achieve greatness, you just cannot give up on that. Know in faith that you will achieve it. Don't listen to the 'naysayers,' just go with your gut and follow your heart.

If you give up and you quit, that's it. It's game over. But if you get knocked down, eventually you will find the strength to GET BACK UP and keep moving. Now that is true power! That is the determination of keeping going and striving for what you want, despite the challenges you may face. It is ok to try and sometimes fail. Failing forward is one of the most profound quotes I've heard from Sir Richard Branson *(previously quoted in the book)* He said, *'If a baby is starting to walk and it falls, is it going to give up? No chance. That baby is going to get up again and keep trying until eventually it is able to walk.'* What an incredible analogy on the perseverance of life.

It's the same with your attitude, mindset and emotional strength that you need to keep moving forward, to achieve success. So please, if anybody is down your throat, feeding you with doubt, you look them straight in the eyes and say to them, *"I'm doing this!"* You don't have to be rude, just say *"I know you care about me and I respect that. But I'm going to keep doing this because I know in my heart that this is the right thing for me to do."*

If you were towards the end of a college degree and things got tough, do you think anybody is going to tell you to give up? Heck No! They're going to tell you to keep working at it because the end is near, and you've worked hard for it; so, why give up now? But, whenever it's a self-pursuing goal that we have, which is different to what everybody else is doing around you, they are more likely going to tell you to stop, because they are unfamiliar with the pursuit. It's not their fault, they just won't have the mindset that you have; therefore, it's unlikely that they will understand. Keep pursuing, and NEVER EVER give up. You've only got one life on this planet, so you might as well make good use of it. You have greatness in you to pursue and achieve your goals and dreams.

Now is the Time!

If you have something that you want to achieve, don't wait, act in accordance with the goal and do not procrastinate. Do it now. A good tip is to get at least one thing done today, not tomorrow. You don't have to spend hours on it, unless it's essential. All you have to do is to take some action and do that one thing. If you want to lose weight or work on your health, you could book in with a local gym or make a to-do list of foods to buy or a list of foods that you need to cut out. Just by doing that one thing, you've imple- mented and taken a step. After that, decide and plan the next steps that you need to take. If it is regarding your relationships and you know you need to talk to your partner, kids or loved ones, perhaps send them a message to start the process of a face-to-face conversation.

If it is your income, create a financial plan of where you would like to be in so many months' time or contact the bank to discuss financial arrangements. If it is a debt related issue, then research and seek advice for a debt management plan. This will take off the stress and pressure like being released from shackles. It might be a business deal and you have to make a list of phones call in order to gain the sale. Out of that list, one of those phone calls could change everything. It all starts with taking that first action. Not tomorrow, not next week or next month, do it TODAY! Do it now! One of the worst things that can happen to you in life is having regret. As I've already said a few times in this book, 'you can always have more things in life, but there's one thing you can't get back and that's more time.' Regret can stay with you for years if you allow it to, but at the end of the day, it is in the past and you can only move forward. There is nobody else to blame but yourself for regret. However, if you have experienced regret, don't beat yourself up because there is a brighter side; it is never too late to make things better.

Have a good think about some of the action plans that you can put into place, and where you want to arrive. Don't think too much about what it will cost you to do it; rather, think more of what it will cost you if you don't. Make sure you implement those actions now. When is the right time? Now, is the time!

Learn how to utilise the formula for the speed of implementation, visit www.changeitbook.com

No Pain, No Gain, No Change

Shortly down the line after some major shifts of change in my life, and the breakthrough realisation about how others had influenced my thinking, attitude and habits, I had landed the perfect marketing job . . . . or, so I thought. I worked extremely hard by always putting the hours in, showing up early and going home late, despite the 1 hour 10-minute journey each day. I always did more than I was asked to do, because I had a real passion for marketing, and really wanted to have an impact on the business.

As the weeks went by, I felt myself growing into the role and became more popular for my work with the senior management. I would take on multiple tasks and do the best I could, and when it was required, I asked for help. Everything was good, which felt like I was doing all the right things. This felt like a dream come true, especially after the hardship in my previous career. I thought I had nailed it. This was a job I had always really wanted since I left the university. This was a new start for me. Finally, things were working out.

After a few months had passed, I had my first review. Whilst I thought I had been performing above and beyond what was expected of me, management had other views and thought I was lacking in certain areas. This was a major shock after all my hard work, and I went from having high self-esteem with a flow of positivity to a feeling of being pushed off a one hundred storey building. Not long after the company decided to let me go.

I soon realised afterwards that I was not meant to stay with this employer, but to move forward for better opportunities. Had I not gone through this experience, I would have not been able to move on and grow further. As a result of my (so called) failures, I managed to increase my income by £10,000 in a short space of time.

'When you hit rock bottom, there is only one way you can go . . . UP!'

Just because someone makes a wrong judgment of you, this does not mean it is true. After the loss of that job, I have realised that if I don't go through these experiences of pain, I can't learn and grow from them. If you have gone through an experience of pain, you can rise again to become a better and stronger person. You must learn from it and never let the experience break you permanently. When you get knocked down, do what you can with what you have, to summon the strength to get back up and rise to a place of accomplishment. If I would have stayed in that job, I would have continued to earn much less along with the pressures and feelings of discouragement. Without the setback, it would have not allowed me to turn my failures into new successes by being pushed into the unknown and taking another leap.

The lesson here is that, you must not see failure as a bad thing, it is a part of life. The experiences are a schooling for greater things in life and are just simple parts of the complexed processes. So, please don't spend too much time blaming others or beating yourself up, when you go through a rough patch. When things go wrong, don't allow your mind to go with them. This example shows that without pain, there is no new opportunity for gain, and without gain, there is no alert for change. Especially when it comes to your income and your self-esteem.

STEP 8

Time:
Don't Waste It!

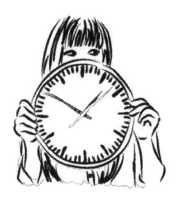

Time Management

The difference between those who are successful (in whatever area or parts of life) and those who are not will depend on how they spend their time. Whether you are a male or a female, young or old, rich or poor, we all have 24 hours in a day. It is the same for everybody. However, how you spend your time within those hours makes all of the difference in how your life turns out.

If we all have an equal amount of time, how can we utilise

the time to gain maximum benefit, so that we don't waste it? Time Management!

Here is the 'Time Management Quadrant' by Dr Stephen Covey, previously mentioned in Step 4 *(Money verses Time)*. Let me try to explain the concept of this model, so you can perhaps identify where it may apply in areas of your life.

Quadrant One, The 'Crisis': it is important and urgent and you must attend to it immediately.

Quadrant Two, The 'Goals': it is not urgent, but is important; we know that it can wait but it is very important.

Quadrant Three, The 'Distractions': it is urgent, but not important; these are things that can get in the way and steer you off focus.

Quadrant Four, A 'Complete Waste of Time': it is not urgent and not important; those are things that are just time-wasting tasks and are side-tracking you from the things that you need to do.

Time Management Quadrant

URGENT & IMPORTANT (CRISIS)	URGENT & NOT IMPORTANT (DISTRACTIONS)
NOT URGENT & IMPORTANT (GOALS) ★	NOT URGENT & NOT IMPORTANT (COMPLETE WASTE OF TIME)

Concept by Dr Stephen R. Covey

Out of the four quadrants, there is only one that is 'key' to unlocking time efficiency and moving you forward for success. That is Quadrant Two: 'Goals.' It is the one that stands out from all the others, to make the most effective use of your time; things that are not urgent, but they are very important. These are the areas in your life that you must work on because that investment in time will drive you forward in the areas of health, relationships and income. All the others are pure distractions, creating barriers in achieving your goals.

I've previously said that you can always get more money, but you can't get more time! How can you invest time in your health? (Mind, body and spirit). How much time is invested in your relationships that count? (Personal, family, and professional relationships). How much time is invested in your income? (Recurring income, savings and investments). Believe it or not, these are very important questions to ask in determining how your life turns out. If you reflect over the last few years and look back at how your life has developed, how have you invested time in the areas of your life, in correlation to the Time Management Quadrant?

First, start with any of the major events that have occurred, whether they are painful or not, just to dig deeper into your time management. Look at the main activities that come to mind on a monthly basis. Then, think about the weekly tasks of where your time has mostly been spent. Finally, look at your daily routines. If you look back at this to see where most of the time has been spent, you will probably say, 'working,' followed by 'spending time taking care of loved ones' (including pets). Around those times there will be relaxing, hobbies, sleeping and let's not forget to mention the time spent scrolling through Facebook.

This is the world we live in; we become so consumed with the day-to-day, trying to multi-task so that we lose track of the bigger picture, and then time just slips through our fingers. But with the use of good time management and setting goals, what can you do to change your schedules to make it work for you? Don't think of the small things; look at the pockets of time that can be implemented to grow into bigger and more significant positive changes. Set goals for the next three months, six months or year. Think about what you could achieve in the next two, five or ten years' time. What can you invest your time in now that's going to make all of the difference in the long run? Start by sketching out a plan and a deadline for a goal, and work backwards to dissect the time frame. Schedule some allocated time and stick to it. Refer to the Time Management Quadrant to check if the time invested in the activities was in good use or just wasted. From time to time you can ask yourself "What quadrant am I in right now?" This focus could prevent you from procrastination and save valuable time being neglected. Reflect on your goals often, and measure the progress being made. The tiny steps that you take to utilise your time will have maximum impact for the better. Now that you have a time management strategy plan, try not to neglect it. Time is most precious, don't waste it.

Is Your Time Used Effectively?

How is most of your time used? What does your weekly schedule look like? And most importantly, is it been used effectively? Time is going way too fast for my liking, quicker than ever before. The advancements of technology and the added pressures that we place upon ourselves due to a fast-paced society can allow us to be consumed by it, to the point of losing a sense of time with the things that count the most, including our joy for others' and our own well-being to create happiness and joy.

When I was much younger as a kid, the time felt like it lasted forever when I was bored, but passed by in the blink of an eye when I was having fun. As I got older and became indulged in modern life by taking on more responsibility, it seems that time is just going by far too quickly. As the months and the years go by, I often have to question if I have used my time effectively to work towards my goals. If not, I then ask myself "How can I be smarter with my time that will have a greater impact?" That's when I then refer to the Time Management Quadrant.

As each new year starts, it is like a starting pistol has gone off, for a 100 meter sprint. Before you know it, two months have passed, then it is spring and onto summer. Then sooner or later it is autumn and then Christmas is here again. We seem to have less time as each year passes and have to work against time, due to the ever-increasing speed. If you value time, then utilising it to its fullest potential will make all the difference to how your life turns out. Focus on the things that are 'not urgent, but important' and do not neglect them.

If it is your health you wish to work on, use the 'eat an apple a day' analogy and embed that principle into your diary for allocated time. This could be done by either identifying the core issues and working on a plan or seeking help from a specialist. Set the goal, don't neglect it, and stick to it!

Now, let's look at your relationships; how much time is invested in 'positive communication' with your loved ones? Listening more than talking, remembering you have two ears and one mouth. I've made countless mistakes in relationships where I've even not listened or have not had the guts to open my mouth, and honestly say deep down 'this is what's wrong.' I have a great relationship now with my daughter, because I've learned from my experiences of lack of communication. I always want to listen to her, and I always ask her questions, rather than just assuming what she wants or wants to do. This can also work really well with professional relationships. As the inspirational speaker and author Simon Sinek would say, "Be the last person to speak in the room." When you spend more time listening to people, and then respond by asking questions, it makes it so much easier to become a good listener, which people will respect more.

Time invested in your income, 'The Big One'. If you're constantly spending your money, do you pay much attention to the habit? This is so easy to neglect. Most people will invest for today rather than the future. Savings are good to have, but investments are even greater. In the last few years, my dad has taught me the value of investing my time by investing my money. He has used this philosophy for fifty years, and because of that, he now has no worries about money. Wouldn't that be great if we could all feel like that? You're damn right it would! Premium bonds, stocks and shares, property or businesses are good ways to invest, but like all investments there are risks, so make sure you do some thorough research and seek trustworthy advice. So, what can you do to balance your spending habits, by retaining more for a greater gain? Think more of how much you can keep, and then how you can perhaps invest to reap the rewards.

Why Now and Not Tomorrow?

The people who really want to make things change for them take immediate action. They don't hesitate. They don't think. They want things to change so they take massive, determined action, and implement it straight away. That's why often wealthy people are wealthy, because they take action and make good use of their time. They don't wait for things to be aligned, for it to be perfect. They start and then perhaps make adjustments along the way, if required. The point is, if you wait and procrastinate, time ends up becoming wasted. It is not about having things perfect, yes we want to do things right for things to turn out well; unfortunately, there is never a perfect time.

By taking action (today and not tomorrow attitude), you get more things done and learn more by doing things quickly. Win/Win. For some tasks, this is by no means easy to get done straight away or reap the results that you want, but you learn from it and then move forward. Implementing that time now can have more of an impact later and perhaps give you more chunks of time.

Let's say that somebody wanted to move into a new job but didn't have the motivation or the courage to do something about it. They wait and wait, the months go by, and before they realise how much time has passed, it is three to four years down the line. They watched others around them move forward with their lives and things just seem to go their way. The successful ones acted and made those choices. For those who didn't, well, let's just say they should be kicking themselves . . . but not too hard. Can you see the significance in the scenarios?

I remember a few years back, I had a conversation with a colleague when I was a teacher in a high school. We were discussing the complexity of the job, and had a small debate on the possibilities of an alternative. She said, "I would love to change my career but I will never be able to find a career that pays me the same salary." At that moment, I said to myself "I have to get out, I have to make a change and I WILL match my income in another field!" That's when I decided to leave the profession, and not long after that conversation, I got the hell out of there.

In her mind, I could sense that she felt stuck where she was and had no plans to come out of the profession. At that point, I decided there and then that wasn't going to be me. I decided to take the hard road of brut action and move on with my life. There is a great book called *The Leap* by Robert Dickie III which focuses on having courage, tenacity and a constructive plan to take the leap into the unknown, rather than waiting for the right time.

Plans are good to have in place, but don't take too long planning or you may procrastinate or talk yourself out of the initial action phase. The action and time invested make all the difference. There is a great saying that I've heard from the renowned motivational speaker Tony Robbins, "It is in the moments of our decisions that our destiny is shaped." If we are all to look back on our lives, we can honestly say that is true.

How Much Time is Left?

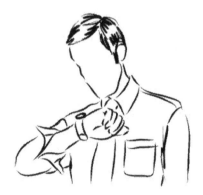

Wherever you are in your life right now, it might be a good idea to calculate how much time you have remaining. This could be for a special occasion, a deadline or a timeframe for a goal. If you can keep track of your time (without having to clock-watch every few minutes) time can work in your favour.

Life can be one big challenge, but many of these challenges are exciting when they are planned correctly. The question is, "How much time do you have left, and what can you do now to make your life better?" I believe that we have choices, and we deserve to live a good life; so, if there are areas in your life that you want to change, then you must take some action now and leap right into it. Don't be that person stuck at the edge of the cliff, waiting for the right time. Be that person who leaps off the cliff knowing that no matter what happens, the parachute will eventually open and will land safely. Things will work out for you. Be determined. Be focused, and have inner self-belief. Be open enough to know that things will turn out for the better in time.

Faith is what has driven me towards my own personal successes, and it will carry on driving me until the day I leave this planet. How much time do I have left, who knows? But, I will make sure that the time I do have left will be maximised on self-growth and helping others do the same. Day by day, keep track of time and due dates of goals, not constantly heading towards burnout, but consistently to make steady progress. Subconsciously think about where you want to go and allow yourself to move towards it in good, measurable time. Beware of others swallowing up your time that is not of value, and try to live the best way that's possible.

We spend so much of our time rushing around, working, earning money and paying bills in order to support families and others, we become guardians, which can lead to neglect of how much time we have left. Now, I just want you to think about that for a few seconds to process this, especially if the above highly resonates with you. Please embed this in your mind to recognise that whatever has happened to you in the past, you can't change it. However, TODAY, you can start a new thought process that can determine your future. I don't mean to scare you; as that is not the aim here. This is merely a jolt in your thinking to identify how precious life is.

Time for Yourself

Countless times over the last few years, I have been running at 100 miles an hour without stopping. When you do that, you end up running on empty and eventually burning out. For me, this was an accumulation of work, being a father, a partner, a good friend, a colleague and a small business owner. Taking on way too much and spinning too many plates can manifest into a burden, by continuing to spin them. We don't realise this at first, but then one by one it becomes an immense weight on our shoulders. Once you hit burn out, you are no good to anyone and then all the plates come crashing down.

I know from my own experiences that when you make time for yourself, you can try to block out the noise of all the spinning plates. Taking 'Adult Timeout' is vital; that bit of space from everything where you can feel at peace, focus on yourself and lay the plates down nicely on the ground. This would be YOUR allocated time to hit the reset button and not process any thoughts for anyone or anything. Not even your loved ones, family, friends, pets or work, just focussing solely on your own well-being. Turn off your phone, TV, laptop, tablet, or any sort of distraction, it needs to be about you and only you. You are more important than you may think. Perhaps, go for a walk or exercise, whether it is in the gym or in a designated place where you can be on your own and have that peaceful space. The aim is to interrupt your thought processes and create a bubble of space by not having to think about other things that are perhaps bothering you in your life right now. You need to separate the reality of what's going on in your busy day-to-day, to just focus on you, be in tune with self. As they say, 'become one.'

Be present in the moment, so there is no worry, stress, anxiety or fear that is attempting to paralyse you. There is nothing but pure PEACE. When you can find a way to practice this and develop more moments for yourself, it can be priceless! This should then start to feed into your neurological brain patterns to convert into new habits, and then manifest into a new belief system. The positive process of this will eventually relieve the bulk of the burdens and stresses. In addition to this newfound principle, take time for yourself to do the things that you love and gives you joy. It will allow you to feel better about yourself, become inspired and motivated in yourself to create and develop new emotions. The happier you feel with more of the smaller things that you do, the more fulfilled you will feel in all that you do.

Find and make time for yourself to block out and minimise the pressures of all the aspects of what's going on in your life. Be at peace with yourself and find things that you love and enjoy doing.

Reflection

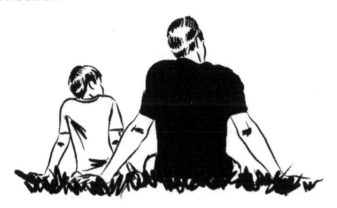

Take a few minutes (right now) to really reflect on your life, currently and previously. Go back as far as you can, to where you were most joyful, happy and content with your life. When you get to that point and identify a 'feeling of abundance,' try to move forward in time to briefly reflect on the elements of your life that have been great and the painful parts that haven't been so good. Then, ask yourself "Was that ok?" The reason I ask you to do this is because it is absolutely one hundred percent crucial that you are deeply honest with yourself, to find out what has been the cause of some of the events that have happened to you during this time, this is the 'cause and effect.' Rather than just focusing on the now and pointing finger at someone else, take some responsibility by looking back at the very start before the experience happened and say, "What could I have done differently?" or "What have I learned from that experience?, so that I know what to expect in the future."

Once you do that, you start to understand the 'cause' to prevent the 'effect' and things will start to make sense to you. Steve Jobs once said, "It's not just about how you move forward, sometimes you have to connect the dots by working backwards, to allow you to understand the bigger picture." Wow! If you can identify the major chain of events that have occurred in your life so far by looking into the cause and then the overall result of how you have ended up where you are today, this may trigger an awakening of realisation. If there are any choices that you may have made in the past and now feel some regret for, please do not dwell on them. Don't feel guilty, and don't be hard on yourself. You can still change the future, but you can't change the past. Think of a way you could learn from that and move forward. The moments of sheer and utter disgust, where you have wanted to give in are the most significant points in your life which have forced you to move forward. Use it as an experience so that you can now learn and implement new ways of how you can make change for the better.

'It's not what happens to you that determines your future; it's what you DO with what happens to you.'
                                                    - Jim Rohn

Whatever experiences you have had, turn them around to make positive change for the future. I want you to say to yourself, "I know I have had some challenges in my life. I know that it hasn't been easy. But from today, I want to make positive transformations and I will make sure that I work towards a better future, because I deserve a good life."

Revelation - Part One

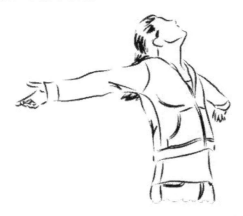

I just want to take a moment to congratulate you for reading this far, well done! Feeding your mind with new profound knowledge and concepts is not always the easiest of tasks to consume straight away. That's why I have broken it down into smaller chunks, so you can feast on it and refer to the pages when necessary. I've managed to manifest and compound the information together, so you can take this and apply it in your own life, and perhaps create a new journey in your life. Go ahead and give yourself a pat on the back and say, "Yes, I did it!" Give yourself some recognition for this investment in yourself, because the things that you now know from reading this book, most people won't know in a complete lifetime! Shocking I know, but it is the truth. Watching their lives slip away, plodding through life without knowing what they could have achieved or what they could have changed for the better.

Confronting new challenges is an exhilarating experience and the only way is to learn and implement. You may be thinking, "I've gone through many challenges and worked hard, yet why am I still struggling?" The difference is that you have to see the future finished in advanced, and do the uncomfortable until it becomes comfortable. By being self-disciplined day by day you, will make a tremendous difference in how your life turns out. You must find the confidence to act upon the discovery of a journey that you could never find before. Transform your belief system, by practicing the new knowledge within the contents of this book, that will start you on a journey and a growing process, then become fascinated by the results you will enjoy. Along the way, if you wish to take on the revealing concepts that I have shared with you, you will also discover new emotions, whether you try or don't try or believe or don't believe. It is the belief system that drives you forward or leaves you parked at the side of the road.

It is not just about the 'knowing' of the information that counts. As I've said in the previous chapter, it is about IMPLEMENTATION, to use your time and try to discover all that you can do and all that you can have during your own life . . . . notice I said 'own life' and not 'other's lives'. As Henry David Thoreau quoted, *"Go confidently in the direction of your dreams. Live the life you have always imagined."* Construct a concrete commitment to yourself to make a long-term vow that you are going to create change by having a great vision of how your life is going to turn out. Along this road, you will face challenges and setbacks that may feel like quicksand, but each time you overcome them, you will get stronger, smarter, faster and eventually become unstoppable. Be patient and give the process time, because believe me, it is worth it. Day by day, week by week, month by month, even year by year, your efforts will compound, and the positive effects will be astronomical. If you haven't yet heard of the term 'compound,' run an internet search *'penny doubled for 31 days'* I guarantee you will be astonished by the results. This is similar to the principles that will apply in your life, with consistent determination and effort that you apply.

On this unique journey, you will have close friends and family who love you, and want to protect you from the dangers of your new venture. This is because some of these concepts will be completely alien to them and perhaps even a shock. As you go on to pursue the path of abundance, the likelihood is that friends and family could try and talk you out of it. *Crazy, I know!* But it is because in their eyes, they want the best for you and don't want to see you get hurt, or for you to feel the great lashes that comes with failure. The brain is trained for one thing only and that is survival (to protect). On the other hand, the prevention by others can be deemed as a reminder of why they themselves should be taking action, making a change and working towards the brighter side . . . but they don't. This will say more about them than it does about you.

Somehow, through mental and emotional strength combined, with focus and faith, you must break through and see past the naysayers, regardless of what people will say or think of you. It is your life and yours only. You make the choice. You choose the direction you want to go, because only you can do that, nobody else can. During a college lecture, Steve Jobs said "Your time is limited, so don't waste your time living somebody else's dream. Don't let the noise of other's opinions drown out your own inner voice, heart and intuition. This will determine what you really want to become." WOW, what a revelation!

These principles apply to your health, they apply to your relationships and they apply to your finances; same principles, just different goals. Anybody can have goals that can be achieved once worked upon. You've just got to work towards them and have belief and faith that they will appear. Live the life that you choose.

Revelation - Part Two

As we draw to a close, I want you to take a minute to look at your life. Have you got all that you've wanted out of it, or has there been some deadweight that you've needed to unload that is affecting your health, relationships or your income? Has your life been inspiring, or has it been debilitating? If so, what fear is in your life that has prevented you to move forward? Be honest, as that's the only way to really identify the truth. What things are causing you the most pain and stopping you from your development? If you can source these gremlins, write each one of them down, and take a good look at them, see which ones stand out and are causing the most pain. Then, you MUST confront them. Confront them, and find a way to work on them to make positive change. This can be one of the hardest things to do, but unless you do it, not much will change. You've heard the saying 'old habits die hard,' use some of the strategies in the previous chapters to help as a starting point. Use this book for support. It is purely down to taking actions for change to allow positive transformations, and only you can make that decision and only you can take that action.

Let's look at the positive part of you; what gifts do you have that bring out the best in you? Whatever they may be, use them to find that inner strength and fortitude to increase your self-esteem, and build on your amazing character. Also, what are some of the things that will give you great self-satisfaction? Things that will make you feel incredible; things that make you feel like you can do anything? Once you have a fulfilled mind, along with a bold attitude, inner strength and faith in yourself, you will be unstoppable. Once you have that, hold on to it and embrace it through your inner courage. Courage is doing what feels right despite your fears, doubts, worries, anxieties and all the challenges that you may have ahead. The most important question to ask yourself is, "Is what you're doing right now giving you what you want?" If not, you need to find that inner courage to confront the fear. Focus on the benefits of taking the leap, taking chances and moving forward, having an aspiring attitude that can produce good health, positive relationships and a good stable income.

When I have taken leaps in the past, even when they were the hardest and difficult times of my life (some terrifying), I can honestly say that I look back now and think, "Wow, I did it." Even when it was difficult a time, made some mistakes and got caught in the mud, I can honestly say "I took that leap and look at where I am now." Don't let the fear immobilise you, if you are not getting what you want. Thinking about it is the difficult part, but you OWE IT TO YOURSELF more than anything. Most people will resist change, they will even fight change, as if the change will be worse than what they are experiencing right now. They are not willing to step out into the unknown and take the chance. You have a great gift, and you have inner creativeness to do the most amazing things on this earth. If you take the chance, you will realise that things will work out for you. It always will, because the universe and God are on your side. Will it be Easy? No. Will it be Rocky? Yes. Will you make some mistakes along the way? Yes. Will you get hurt and feel some emotional pain? Yes . . . But is it WORTH IT? ...YES! YES! YES!

Learn how to effectively manage your time for maximum impact, visit www.changeitbook.com

Revelation - Part Three

Now that you have looked back at your life, you have probably identified revealing truths, and it may have been hard for you to do that. You have possibly been shocked by some of the pain that you have experienced through your life, and in some cases, you may have stumbled across the pain of regret, because you know you cannot change the past and often wish you could go back and do things differently. But here's the thing, you can't change the past, but you can change your future. If it has been a painful experience for you to dig deep to core roots, I just want to say 'Let It Go,' to release and increase the peace.

If you look towards your future and what you want to become, to achieve joy, happiness, health, wealth and greatness, it is going to take EVERYTHING in YOU to manifest what you deserve.

If you hear that self-doubt in your mind, trying to tell you that you are not good enough in whatever you are trying to achieve (health, relationships, income) please ignore that voice trying to talk you out of it. Give that part what I like to call the 'Ego Elbow' and say Get Lost! Just focus on and listen to your inner voice, and that inner gut feeling which comes from the heart. Once you have got past that, as you start to work on making positive transformations, you will start to see opportunities open up for you. Good things will start being attracted to you. Even good people will start being attracted to you.

Your creativeness will start to come out, and the new ideas for yourself will appear in front of you as you begin to focus on them more. Keep hold of that vision, focus and faith, and never let go; this is your 'inner treasure,' your ticket to a better life. Picture this, a ball being clenched by a sportsman in a tough brutal contact sport such as the NFL; the same rules apply for your inner treasure. Never ever give up trying along the journey of mystery and complexity to the transformational life change. As you proceed, make sure that you do all that you can to achieve what you truly deserve. Life is not a walk in the park, it is hard; so, make a commitment to yourself. As you look and focus towards your future, know that it is all worth it in the end. Your life is worth it!

From this day forward, I want you to make a contribution to your life and possibly the lives of others in the future. I believe you have a great gift. I believe there is inner great -ness and courage within you. I BELIEVE IN YOU!

I wish you the best of luck in whatever journey you take. But remember, you have choices. You've only got ONE life, so make it a **Good One**.

Are you ready to make positive transformation in your life? Start now by visiting my website
www.changeitbook.com

'If YOU want things to IMPROVE,
YOU must IMPROVE.

If YOU want things to get BETTER,
YOU must get BETTER.

For things to CHANGE, YOU must CHANGE,

. . . and when YOU CHANGE,

EVERYTHING CHANGES for YOU.'

—Jim Rohn

Bibliography

Books:

Live Your Dreams, Les Brown

The Answer, John Asaraf

How to Win Friends and Influence people, Dale Carnegie

Rich Dad Poor Dad, Robert Kiyosaki

Beach Money, Jordan Adler

Passion into Profit: How to Make Big Money from Who You Are and What You Know, Andy Harrington

The Slight Edge, Jeff Olsen

The Secret, Rhonda Byrne

Feel the Fear and Do It Anyway, Susan Jeffers

No Excuse: The Power of Self Discipline, Brian Tracy

Master Your Wow, Vishal Morjaria

Audiobooks:

Challenge to Succeed, Jim Rohn

Awaken the Giant, Tony Robbins

67 Steps, Tai Lopez

Project Life Mastery, Stefan James

The 7 Habits of Highly Effective People, Dr. Stephen Covey

Secrets of a Millionaire Mind, T. Harv Eker

The Success Principles, Jack Canfield

The Leap, Robert Dickie III

Bonus Material: Visit www.changeitbook.com

- Videos on tips and strategies for a positive life, and self-transformation
- Videos on stories relating to positive self-transformation and dealing with day-to-day problems
- Resources for personal development and income strategies
- Downloadable documents to aid positive life transformation
- Blog content on life transformation and stories

Profiles:

Website – www.changeitbook.com

Facebook – facebook.com/groups/discouragementinto recognition

Instagram – c.j.alexander

Twitter – cj xander @dirmotiv8

YouTube – Discouragement into Recognition

Printed in Great Britain
by Amazon